Clinical Cases in Dermatology

Series Editor

Robert A. Norman
Tampa, FL, USA

This series of concise practical guides is designed to facilitate the clinical decision-making process by reviewing a number of cases and defining the various diagnostic and management decisions open to clinicians.

Each title is illustrated and diverse in scope, enabling the reader to obtain relevant clinical information regarding both standard and unusual cases in a rapid, easy to digest format. Each focuses on one disease or patient group, and includes common cases to allow readers to know they are doing things right if they follow the case guidelines.

More information about this series at http://www.springer.com/series/10473

Sunil Kothiwala
Anup Kumar Tiwary
Piyush Kumar
Editors

Clinical Cases in Disorders of Melanocytes

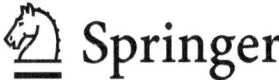 Springer

Editors
Sunil Kothiwala
SkinEva Clinic
Jaipur
India

Anup Kumar Tiwary
Department of Dermatology
Subharti Medical College
Meerut, Uttar Pradesh
India

Piyush Kumar
Katihar Medical College and
Hospital
Bihar
India

Clinical Cases in Dermatology
ISBN 978-3-030-22756-2   ISBN 978-3-030-22757-9   (eBook)
https://doi.org/10.1007/978-3-030-22757-9

This Springer imprint is published by the registered company Springer Nature Switzerland AG
The registered company address is: Gewerbestrasse 11, 6330 Cham, Switzerland

Preface

The study of pigmentary disorders has attracted a lot of attention in the recent past. The extent of disease and the psychological impact of different pigmentary disorders such as vitiligo, melasma and lichen planus pigmentosus can be severe, more so in people with coloured skin. Social stigma and discrimination too are known and can be devastating for the affected patients. Treatment of various conditions presenting with dyspigmentation remains challenging, and improving the quality of life of patients suffering from such conditions is another important treatment goal. While some diseases are restricted to skin and mucosa only, others are visible manifestations of underlying systemic diseases. Dermatologists and physicians should be able to recognize pigmentary changes related to various systemic diseases in order to provide better and timely care to the patient.

Melanocytes are derived from the neural crest cells and after extensive migration during development, they finally reside in skin, inner ear, and uveal tract as highly dendritic, heavily pigmented cells. These cells synthesize melanin within melanosomes which get transferred to neighbouring keratinocytes. Any abnormality in migration from neural crest, melanin synthesis or transfer of melanosomes to keratinocytes may result in melanocytic disorders manifesting as altered pigmentation. Additionally, melanocytes assume crucial roles in inner ear and uveal tract, evident as the presence of ocular and hearing symptoms in many melanocytic disorders.

This book does not attempt to cover all melanocytic disorders but focuses on common pigmentary disorders which clinicians see in their routine practise. The chapters start with a representative case, followed by a discussion on aetiopathogenesis, diagnostic methods and treatment modalities of various hyperpigmentary and hypopigmentary disorders. The format, established by series editor Robert A Norman, provides a quick, easy to digest review of different conditions. We hope that this work will be helpful to young as well as experienced clinicians who have interest in melanocytic disorders.

Jaipur, India   Sunil K. Kothiwala
Uttar Pradesh, India   Anup Kumar Tiwary
Bihar, India   Piyush Kumar

Acknowledgements

We express our gratitude to the authors for working tirelessly on this project and completing the chapters on time.

We are grateful to our teachers for showing us the path.

We thank all our patients, who kept faith in us and taught us a lot.

We thank all our students, past and present: we learn more when we teach.

We are thankful to the Springer staff for doing an excellent job in making this book project a success.

Contents

Contributors

Dipak Kumar Agarwalla, MD Gauhati Medical College and Hospital, Guwahati, India

Ashi, MD Dermatologist, Sadar Hospital, Supaul, Bihar, India

P. C. Das, MD Apoorva Skin Centre, Katihar, India

Subhash Dasarathan, DVD College of Medicine and JNM Hospital, Kalyani, India

Panchami Debbarman, MD Consultant Dermatologist, Mumbai, India

Gunjan Jha, DNB Department of Internal Medicine, Fortis Hospital, Noida, India

Sunil Kumar Kothiwala, MD Dr Kothiwala's SkinEva Clinic, Jaipur, India

Dhiraj Kumar, MD All India Institute of Medical Sciences, Patna, India

Pawan Kumar, MD Kempegowda Institute of Medical Sciences, Bengaluru, India

Piyush Kumar, MD Katihar Medical College and Hospital, Katihar, India

Niharika Ranjan Lal ESI PGIMSR and ESI Medical College, Kolkata, India

Rajesh Kumar Mandal, MD North Bengal Medical College, Darjeeling, India

Avijit Mondal, MD College of Medicine and JNM Hospital, Kalyani, India

Pooja Nupur, MD Nalanda Medical College and Hospital, Patna, India

Swetalina Pradhan, MD All India Institute of Medical Sciences, Patna, India

Divya Sachdev, DDVL Consultant Dermatologist, Raipur, India

Kananbala Sahu, MD All India Institute of Medical Sciences, Bhubaneswar, India

Preeti Sharma, MD All India Institute of Medical Sciences, Patna, India

Anup Kumar Tiwary, MD Department of Dermatology, Subharti Medical College, Meerut, Uttar Pradesh, India

Md. Zeeshan, MD Patna Medical College and Hospital, Patna, India

Part I
Developmental/Migration Disorders

Chapter 1
Bluish Gray Pigmented Macule on Right Cheek

Sunil Kumar Kothiwala

A 22 years old male patient presented with single hyperpigmented macule on left cheek. Patient noticed initial lesion in form of asymptomatic hyperpigmented macule at age of 12–13 years, which gradually increased in size and darken in color but now since last 1–2 years it is stable. He had not taken any treatment for this and the family history was also non-contributory. On examination there was single unilateral blue-to-gray speckled or mottled coalescing smooth surfaced patch involving malar and forehead area of left side of face. Slight pigmentation of the ipsilateral nasal ala was appreciable. Ocular examination showed involvement of sclera in form of grey-blue pigmentation (Fig. 1.1). Oral cavity was not involved.

Based on this clinical information what is your diagnosis?

(a) Spilus nevus
(b) Nevus of Ota
(c) Café-au-lait macule
(d) Segmental lentigenosis

Histopathology showed elongated dendritic melanocytes around collagen bundles in superficial dermis.

S. K. Kothiwala (✉)
Dr Kothiwala's SkinEva Clinic, Jaipur, India

© Springer Nature Switzerland AG 2020   3
S. Kothiwala et al. (eds.), *Clinical Cases in Disorders of Melanocytes*, Clinical Cases in Dermatology,
https://doi.org/10.1007/978-3-030-22757-9_1

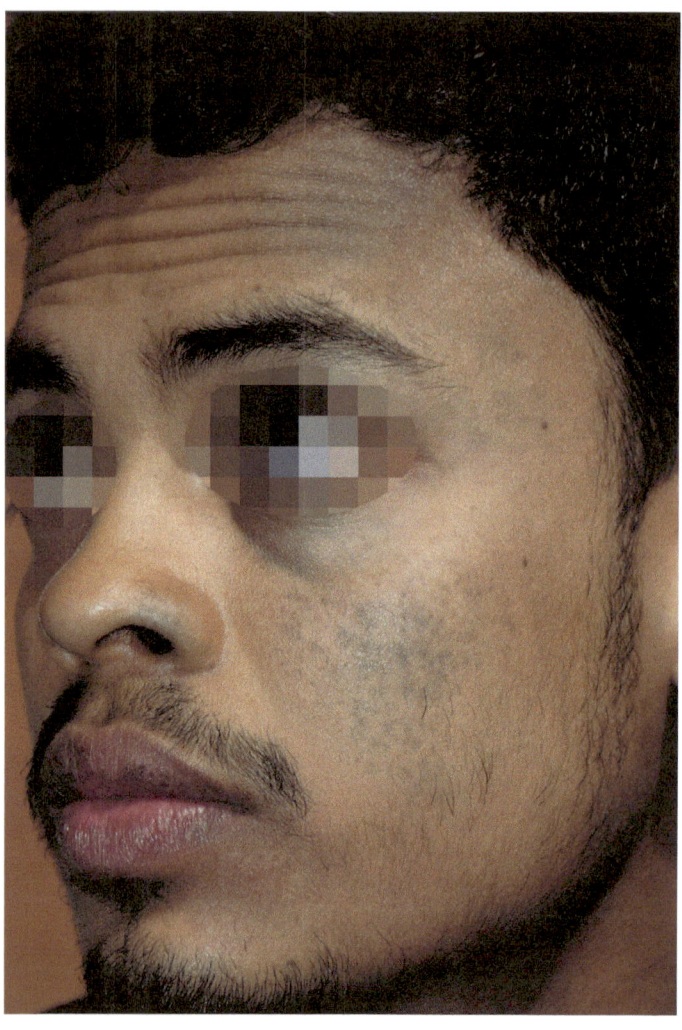

FIGURE 1.1 Young male is having bluish colored large macule on left cheek with scleral involvement

Diagnosis

• Nevus of Ota

Discussion

Nevus of Ota is a type of dermal melanocytosis characterized by unilateral bluish gray mottled pigmented macule with or without extracutaneous involvement. Histopathology shows dermal dendritic melanocytes deep within dermis. Various treatment modalities including lights and lasers had been tried with variable success.

During fetal development, normally melanocytes migrate from the neural crest to the dermal-epidermal junction (DEJ). However, these melanocytes may occasionally fail to reach at DEJ and remain entrapped in dermis where due to Tyndall effect brown color of these nevus cells give bluish gray color to skin surface. Exact etiology is not known but specific mutations have been detected within the dermal melanocytes, most often GNAQ or GNA11 suggesting a link between nevus of Ota and uveal melanoma. Several theories have been put forward which include: dropping-off of epidermal melanocytes, migration of hair bulb melanocytes, reactivation of pre-existing latent dermal melanocytes, which are triggered by dermal inflammation, UV radiation or hormonal changes during pregnancy [1].

There are four types of dermal melanocytosis: nevus of Ota, nevus of Ito, nevus of hori, and Mongolian spot (Table 1.1).

Nevus of ota usually occurs in Asian populations with an incidence between 0.014 and 0.034% and especially common in Japanese [2]. It is more frequent in females. It has two peak ages of onset at birth or early infancy and in early adolescence. It also known as nevus fuscoceruleus ophthalmomaxillaris or oculodermal melanocytosis as clinical presentation follows distribution of ophthalmic and maxillary divisions of the trigeminal nerve.

TABLE 1.1 Different types of dermal melanocytosis

Type	Epidemiology	Onset	Clinical	Distribution	Histopathology	Associated features
Nevus of Ota	Asian (Japanese), female	Early infancy or adolescent	Blue-gray speckled pigmentation	In distribution of ophthalmic and maxillary branches of trigeminal nerve	Elongated dendritic dermal melanocytes in dermis	Glaucoma Ocular melanoma Has been reported with Neurofibromatosis type 1
Nevus of Ito	Asian and female	Early infancy or adolescent	Blue-gray speckled pigmentation	In distribution of Acromioclavicular nerve	Elongated dendritic dermal melanocytes in dermis	None
Mongolian spot	Asian, African and male	At birth or within first few weeks	Blue-gray uniform pigmentation	Lower back, sacral region	Spindle shaped dendritic melanocytes in deep dermis	Usually resolve within 1 year Extra sacral lesions tend to persist more than 1 year Persistent Mongolian spots are associated with inborn error of metabolism
Nevus of hori	Asian and female	Second to fourth decade	Blue-gray speckled pigmentation	Area similar to nevus of ota but bilateral involvement	Elongated dendritic dermal melanocytes in dermis	None
Dermal melanocytic hamartoma		Congenital	Blue-gray speckled macules in a diffuse pigmented patch	Dermatomal	Dermal melanocytes in upper second/third dermis	None

Tanino has classified it in four classes based on distribution of lesion: [3]

- Type I. Mild type
  - IA. Mild orbital type: Distribution over the upper and lower eyelids, periocular and temple region.
  - IB. Mild zygomatic type: Pigmentation is found in the infrapalpebral fold, nasolabial fold and the zygomatic region.
  - IC. Mild forehead type: Involvement of the forehead alone.
  - ID. Involvement of alanasi alone.
- Type II. Moderate type: Distribution over the upper and lower eyelids, periocular, zygomatic, cheek and temple regions.
- Type III. The lesion involves the scalp, forehead, eyebrow and nose.
- Type IV. Bilateral type: Both sides are involved.

Clinically it is characterized by speckled or mottled blue gray or brown or mixed pigmented coalescing macules or patches involving periorbital region, malar area, temple, forehead and nose. Most cases are unilateral but can be bilateral. Ocular involvement is next common site to skin in which the sclera and the bulbar and palpebral conjunctiva are most commonly affected. Glaucoma and ocular melanoma are rare complications. Oral lesions involving buccal mucosa or palate have been reported. Exogenous factors like Emotions, fatigue, insomnia, unusually warm or cold weather may increase the colour tone. Hormonal fluctuations associated with menses and menopause can also cause darkening of the lesion [4].

Acquired bilateral nevus of ota like macule (Hori nevus) is located at same skin areas as nevus of Ota without mucosal involvement. It usually develop in second to fourth decade of life and present as bilateral, blue-gray or brown macules or patches.

Common differential diagnosis is hori nevus, nevus spilus, melasma, blue nevus, segmental lentiginosis and café-au-lait macule.

Nevus spilus is black brown or red brown macules within a patch of tan to brown hyperpigmentation. Lesions are usually noted in early infancy and face and trunk are most common sites. It has two different presentations, nevus spilus maculosus and papulosus. Macular form is associated with phacomatosis pigmentovascularis, whereas papular form is with phacomatosis pigmentokeratotica and speckled lentigenous nevus syndrome. Histopathology shows increased pigmentation in basal layer, multiple nests of melanocytes at DEJ in macular form and in dermis in papular form.

Segmental lentiginosis (partial unilateral lentiginosis or agminated lentigines) is an example of cutaneous mosaicism. Clinically it presents with multiple grouped lentigines in segmental pattern with sharp demarcation at mid line. It can occur at any side with slight predilection for face, neck and extrimities. It can be part of neurofibromatosis type 1.

Café-au-lait macules (CALM) are light brown to dark brown colored hyperpigmented lesions which vary in size. Usually it is associated with neurofibromatosis type 1 in 95% of cases, McCune-Albright syndrome, Legius syndrome, tuberous sclerosis and fanconi anemia. It may be observed in infancy in form of very light brown colored macule or patch which gradually become more appreciable. Solitary large CALMs are larger than 0.5 cm and located commonly over buttocks and usually not associated with any syndrome.

Blue nevus is common benign melanocytic nevus with dermal melanocytosis typically present as single dark blue or blue-black dome shaped papule with diameter of less than 1–2 cm. rarely large lesions, ulcerations or subcutaneous nodule, agminate, eruptive and target lesions have also been reported. Most common sites are face, scalp, and dorsum of distal extremities.

The diagnosis of dermal melanocytosis is based on color of lesion and location. In this case, presence of blue-gray color of pigmentation, speckled pattern, unilateral involvement and scleral involvement suggested the diagnosis of nevus of

Ota. Skin biopsy usually required on suspicion of malignant transformation. Ophthalmic examination may be required to rule out any change in intraocular pressure.

Histopathology shows elongated dendritic melanocytes scattered among collagen bundles mainly in the superficial dermis, occasionally they may extend deeper in dermis or subcutaneous tissue. Compared to Mongolian spot, number of melanocytes is much more. Dermal melanophages may be present.

Medical treatment is comprised of cosmetic camouflage to reduce disfigurement due to nevus of ota. Pulsed Q-switched laser (ruby, alexandrite, nd:yag) treatments are first line of treatment for nevi of Ota and Ito. Multiple sessions (4–8) may be required to achieve 90–100% clearance [5]. Other treatment options are cryosurgery, dermabrasion and surgical excision.

Key Points
- Dermal melanocytosis are result of entrapment of migratory melanocytes in dermis during fetal development and usually identified by their blue-gray color and peculiar location.
- Nevus of ota occurs unilaterally and typically involves distribution areas of ophthalmic and maxillary division of trigeminal nerve.
- Hori nevus is different from nevus of ota by presence of lesion bilaterally without mucosa involvement.

Diagnostic Pearls
- Unilateral speckled or mottled blue-gray coalescing macules or patches.
- Sclera or conjunctiva involvement is present in 60% of cases of nevus of Ota.
- Histopathology is characterized by elongated dendritic dermal melanocytes which are more in number than Mongolian spot.

References

1. Stanford DG, Georgouras KE. Dermal melanocytosis: a clinical spectrum. Aust J Dermatol. 1996;37:19–25.
2. Hidano A, Kajima H, Ikeda S, et al. Natural history of nevus of Ota. Arch Dermatol. 1967;95:187–95.
3. Tanino H. Nevus fuscoceruleus ophthalmomaxillaris Ota. Jpn J Dermatol. 1939;46:435–51.
4. Sekar S, Kuruvila M, Pai HS. Nevus of Ota: a series of 15 cases. Indian J Dermatol Venereol Leprol. 2008;74:125–7.
5. Nam JH, Kim HS, Choi YJ, Jung HJ, Kim WS. Treatment and classification of nevus of Ota: a seven-year review of a single institution's experience. Ann Dermatol. 2017;29:446–53.

Part II
Melanocyte Senescence

Chapter 2
Multiple Depigmented Macules on Trunk

Pawan Kumar

A 55 year old male presents with multiple hypopigmented macules over back and abdomen since 1 year. They are asymptomatic and there is no increase in size after onset but they are increasing in number. No other family member is affected. On examination he had multiple small round or angular hypo- and depigmented smooth surfaced macules of size ranging from 1 to 5 mm over abdomen and back (Fig. 2.1). Palm and sole are normal. Based on this clinical information and photograph what is the diagnosis?

(a) Hyperkeratotic confetti leukoderma
(b) Vitiligo
(c) Idiopathic guttate hypomelanosis
(d) Cole's disease

Dermoscopy of largest lesion revealed amoeboid pattern with pseudopod like projections (Fig. 2.2).

Diagnosis

- Idiopathic guttate hypomelanosis

P. Kumar (✉)
Kempegowda Institute of Medical Sciences, Bengaluru, India

© Springer Nature Switzerland AG 2020   13
S. Kothiwala et al. (eds.), *Clinical Cases in Disorders of Melanocytes*, Clinical Cases in Dermatology,
https://doi.org/10.1007/978-3-030-22757-9_2

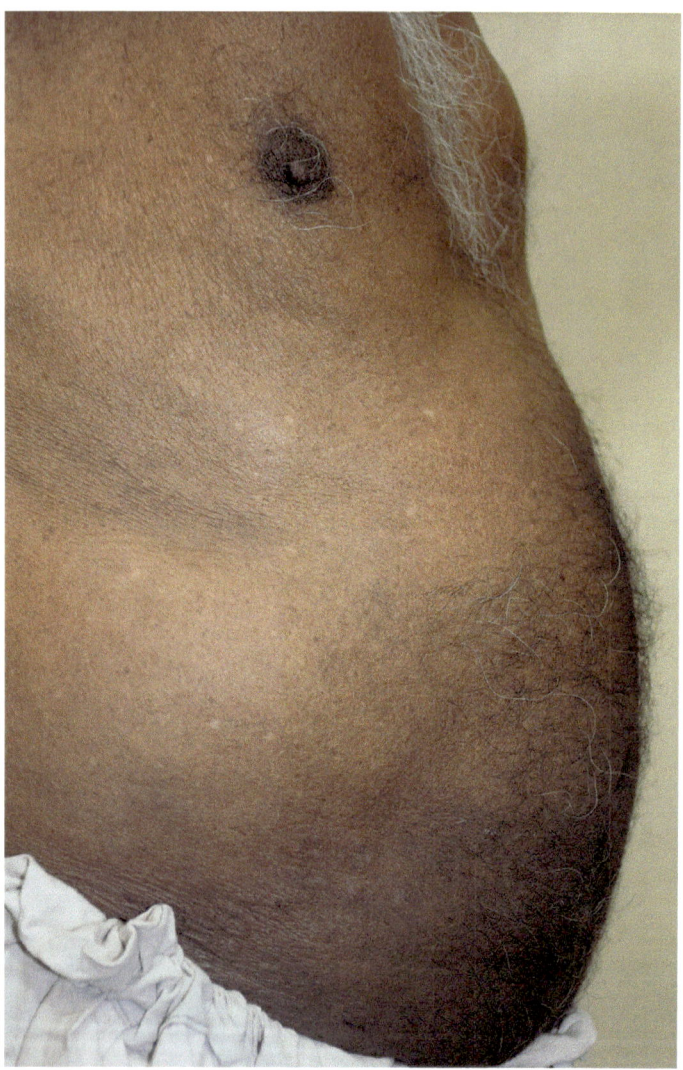

FIGURE 2.1 Multiple depigmented sharply demarcated macule on abdomen and back. (Courtesy: Dr. Piyush Kumar)

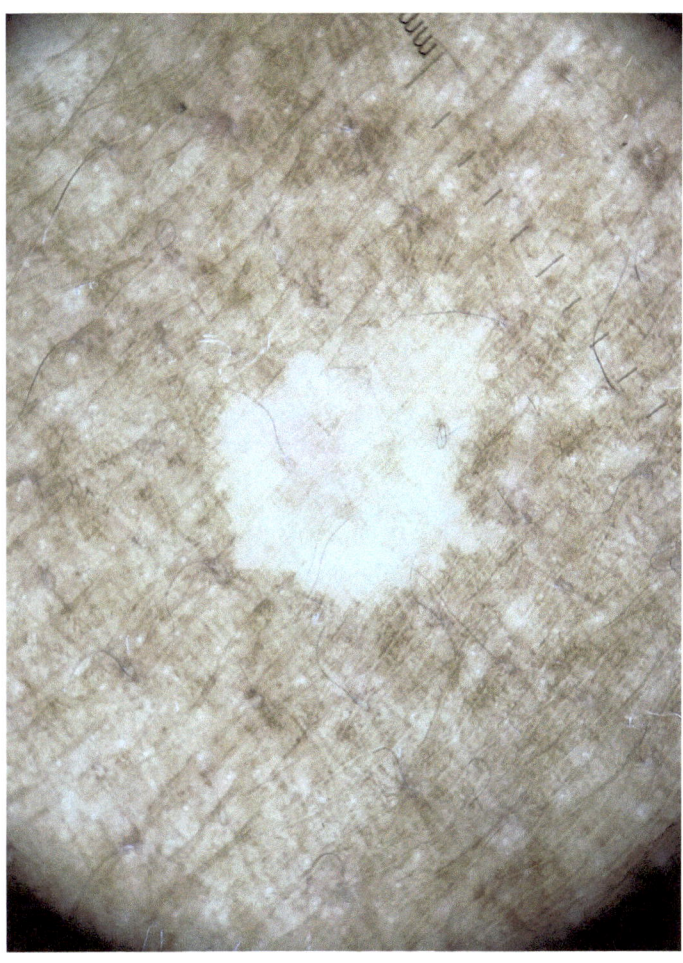

FIGURE 2.2 Dermoscopy image showing amoeboid pattern with pseudopod like projections. (Courtesy: Dr. Piyush Kumar)

Discussion

Idiopathic guttate hypomelanosis (IGH) is a common, acquired and benign dermatosis. The incidence of IGH is associated with advancing age. Although it affects nearly 87% of the population aged more than 40 years, it may also be seen in young adults into the 20s and 30s. Some studies report a female predilection. It is more frequent in fair-skinned people.

Pathogenesis of IGH is not well known. Ageing, chronic sun exposure, genetics, trauma, autoimmunity, and local inhibition of melanogenesis have been proposed as causative factors [1]. Sunlight has been long incriminated in the pathogenesis of IGH because lesions are mainly located at sun exposed body areas, as evidenced by occurrence of IGH lesions in patients receiving PUVA/NB-UVB treatments. Repeated trauma plays a role. High incidence of lesions on the anterior surface of tibias, where subcutaneous tissue is less, and in persons using body scrubs clearly shows that the successional irritation of vulnerable body parts may essentially contribute to the formation of IGH lesions.

Clinically IGH is characterized by multiple, small, scattered, discrete, round or oval, porcelain-white macules ranging in size from 0.2 to 2 cm. They are smooth but occasionally scaling may be present. Skin markings are reduced within lesion. The macules are usually seen in upper and lower extremities, trunk and face. The number increases with time but size remains same. There is no spontaneous repigmentation. Usually they are asymptomatic even though some mention mild itching.

Diagnosis is usually made on clinical grounds. The main histopathological findings observed in IGH lesions are basket weave hyperkeratosis, patchy absence or decreased number of melanocytes and flat rete-ridges [2]. Melanocytes may have less melanosomes, dilatated endoplasmic reticulum, swelled mitochondria and attenuated dendrites. Melanosomes contained in the adjacent keratinocytes may be reduced or even absent. Dermoscopy shows normally pigmented specks scattered within the macules and perimetric pigmentary extensions. IGH may be developed according to four patterns, which are nebuloid, petaloid, amoeboid and feathery. Dermoscopy can be a valuable tool in the evaluation of lesions of IGH [3]. IGH can assume varying morphologies on dermoscopy:

- Amoeboid: most common presentation, pseudopod-like extensions
- Feathery: irregularly pigmented with feathery margins and whitish central area
- Petaloid: polycyclic margins, resembling petals of a flower
- Nebuloid: indistinct, smudged borders. More often in early lesions.

Hyperkeratotic confetti leukoderma presents quite similar to IGH like lesions but they are more uniformly disseminated and lesions have a discrete hyperkeratotic scale. They usually develop after PUVA therapy. Sometimes it has been described as morphological variant of IGH but there are insufficient evidences to describe whether they could share the same pathogenesis.

Vitiligo at early stages needs to be differentiating from IGH especially when lesions are located at shins and forearm. Vitiligo can occur at any site, sometimes it follows trauma (koebners phenomenon). They increase in size with time and spontaneous perifollicular repigmentation is common. Presence of leukotrichia within or in periphery of lesion favors vitiligo over IGH.

Cole's disease is uncommon congenital skin disease with autosomal inheritance. It is characterized by hypomelanotic macules with punctate keratosis of the palms and soles. Immunohistochemistry showed a reduction in the melanin pigment in the keratinocytes and normal pigmentation in the melanocytes which suggests that it is disorder of transfer mechanism of melanosomes from melanocytes to keratinocytes.

Other differential diagnosis are macular hypomelanosis, pityriasis versicolor, tuberous sclerosis, lichen sclerosus et atrophicus, guttate morphea, and post inflammatory hypopigmentation. Macular hypomelanosis have less sharply described lesions. Pityriasis versicolor lesions have fine scale and usually found on upper back, neck and shoulders.

Although treatment is not usually required, the most effective treatment is the careful destruction of the lesion using trichloroacetic acid (TCA) or phenol, cryotherapy, dermabrasion or Fractional co2/erbium yag laser. Spot peel with 88% phenol, repigmentation was observed in 64% of the treated lesions in a study [4]. Cryotherapy works by causing inactivation of inhibitory enzyme or other chemokines participating in melanogenesis and the removal of the defective keratinocytes. It is speculated that the thermal damage, caused by lasers, is the key determinant for the removal of dysfunctional melanocytes and the induction of a healing process which stimulates the secretion of cytokines and growth factors and enhances the recruitment and proliferation of the surrounding melanocytes [5]. Few patients exhibited erythema and post-inflammation hyperpigmentation which are common side effects. Topical retinoids, topical steroids and topical calcineurin inhibitor have also been suggested with variable results.

Key Points

- IGH is very common acquired hypopigmention disorder characterized by small, discrete depigmented macules that usually present after 40 year of age.
- Chronic sun exposure and repetitive minor trauma are believed to be major causing factor.
- Pathologically IGH lesion shows decrease in melanin pigment and number of melanocytes in IGH lesions with skip areas of retained melanin.
- There is no spontaneous repigmentation and they increase in number with age but not in size.

References

1. Juntongjin P, Laosakul K. Idiopathic guttate hypomelanosis: a review of its etiology, pathogenesis, findings, and treatments. Am J Clin Dermatol. 2016;17(4):403–11.
2. Kim SK, Kim EH, Kang HY, Lee ES, Sohn S, Kim YC. Comprehensive understanding of idiopathic guttate hypomelanosis: clinical and histopathological correlation. Int J Dermatol. 2010;49(2):162–6.
3. Ankad BS, Beergouder SL. Dermoscopic evaluation of idiopathic guttate hypomelanosis: a preliminary observation. Indian Dermatol Online J. 2015;6(3):164–7.
4. Ravikiran SP, Sacchidanand S, Leelavathy B. Therapeutic wounding—88% phenol in idiopathic guttate hypomelanosis. Indian Dermatol Online J. 2014;5(1):14–8.
5. Rerknimitr P, Chitvanich S, Pongprutthipan M, Panchaprateep R, Asawanonda P. Non-ablative fractional photothermolysis in treatment of idiopathic guttate hypomelanosis. J Eur Acad Dermatol Venereol. 2015;29(11):2238–42.

Part III
Hypermelanotic Disorders

Chapter 3
Young Female with Multiple Pigmented Macules on Face

Sunil Kumar Kothiwala

A 20 years old female presented with multiple brown pigmented macules over cheek, nose and upper eyelids. Patient noticed these lesions in early childhood which gradually increased in number and intensity of color for next few years. There was no history of spontaneous resolution of lesions. There is no history of any systemic complain. Family history was not contributory. On examination patient had numerous, round to oval shaped dark brown uniformly pigmented discrete macules with irregular margins distributed over face predominantly involving malar area and nose. Some lesions were present on upper eyelids and lower lip (Fig. 3.1). Very few scattered lesions were present over extremities. There was no mucosa involvement.

Based on this information what is your diagnosis?

(a) Freckles
(b) Simple lentigo
(c) Carney complex
(d) Centerofacial lentiginosis

S. K. Kothiwala (✉)
Dr Kothiwala's SkinEva Clinic, Jaipur, India

© Springer Nature Switzerland AG 2020   23
S. Kothiwala et al. (eds.), *Clinical Cases in Disorders of Melanocytes*, Clinical Cases in Dermatology,
https://doi.org/10.1007/978-3-030-22757-9_3

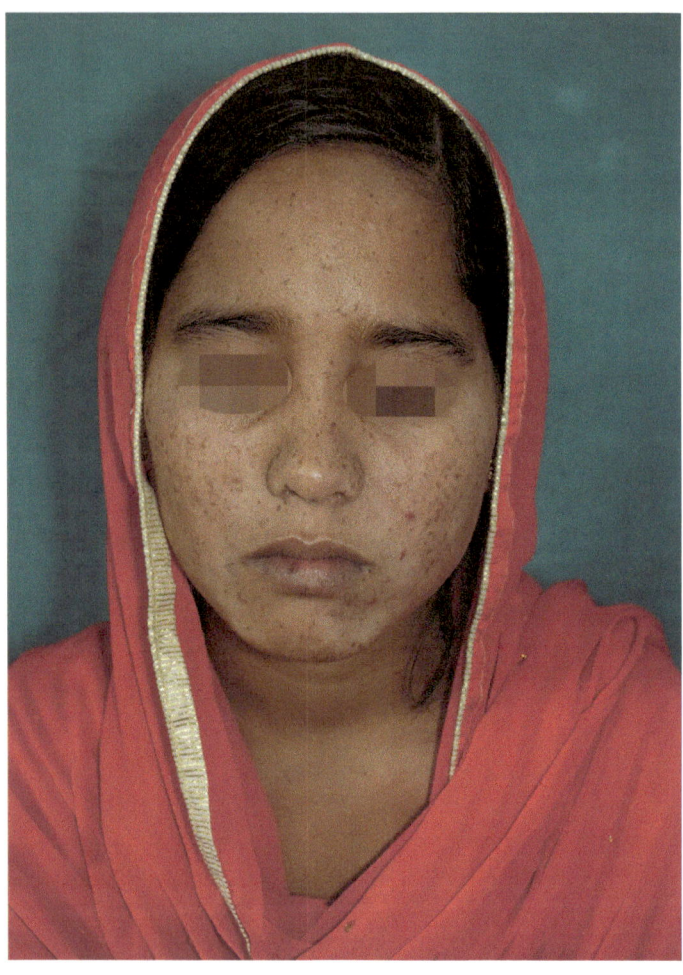

FIGURE 3.1 A young female with multiple discrete dark brown macules over face

Diagnosis

- **Simple lentigo**

Discussion

Lentigines are hyperpigmented macules appearing on normal skin after ultraviolet (UV) rays exposure. There is increased number of melanocytes but not forming nests resulting in hyper pigmentation of basal layer which do not fade away after avoidance of UV exposure. Types of lentigines are: simple lentigo, solar lentigo, psoralene and UVA (PUVA) lentigo and ink-spot lentigo. Rarely, lentigines occur in association with hereditary multisystem syndromes.

Lentigines arise more commonly in light skinned individuals affecting children as well as adult in both sexes. Cause of lentigo depends on its type. Solar and ink-spot lentigo are associated with sun exposure, PUVA lentigo are associated with PUVA therapy and genetic factors are associated with other familial lentiginosis syndromes [1].

Lentigo simplex is the most common lentigo and chronic sun exposure is most important causing factor. Usually it starts in early childhood but sometimes lesions may present at birth or develop later. They gradually increase in number with age. Clinically lesions are round to oval, 3–5 mm in size, brown to black uniformly pigmented macules with jagged or smooth margin. They are asymptomatic and predominantly present over sun-exposure areas but may involve covered areas as well as mucosa without any other systemic involvement. Compared to freckles lentigines are darker in color and comparatively have sparseness in arrangement and scattered distribution. Avoidance of sun-exposure doesn't lead to resolution of lesions [2].

Histopathology of lentigo simplex shows increased pigmentation of basal layer with slight increase in number of non-atypical melanocytes. Dermoscopy shows scalloped borders, pseudonetwork and structureless areas.

Lentigo simplex need to be differentiate from other types of lentigo, familial lentiginosis syndromes, ephelids (freckles), small junctional nevus, flat small seborrhoeic keratosis and lentigomaligna.

Other types of lentigo and familial lentiginosis syndromes have been summarized in Tables 3.1 and 3.2 [3] respectively.

Table 3.1 Types of lentigo

Types	Cause	Onset	Clinical	Distribution
Lentigo simplex	Sun-exposure	Starts in early childhood	Light brown to dark brown uniformly pigmented round to oval macule with jagged/smooth margin	Predominantly photoexposed sites
Solar lentigo	Sun-exposure (chronic or intermittent)	Usually appear in adults	Brown colored large macule with irregular border	Photoexposed sites
PUVA lentigo	PUVA	After high cumulative photochemotherapy More common in men	Large pigmented macule	Sites receiving PUVA
Ink spot lentigo	Sun exposure		Small dark black macules with irregular margin resembling an ink spots	Photoexposed sites

TABLE 3.2 Familial lentiginosis syndromes

Syndrome	Inheritance	Gene	Lentigines	Systemic features
Peutz-Jeghers syndrome	Autosomal dominant	LKB1/STK11 (19p13.3)	Brown-blue macules are commonly found on the border of the lips, oral and bowel mucosa, palms and soles, eyes, nares, and peri-anal region	Gastrointestinal hamartomatous polyps, neoplasm (GI, pancreas, breast, ovary, uterus, testis)
Carney complex	Autosomal dominant	PRKAR1A (17q22-24)	Mucocutaneous lentigines involving inner canthi and genital mucosa Note: freckling, café-au-lait macule and blue nevi may also present	Cardiac and skin myxomas, schwannomas, acromegaly, endocrine, breast and testicular tumor
LEOPARD syndrome	Autosomal dominant	PTPN11 (12q24.1) RAF1 (3p25)	Lentigines mainly involving face and upper trunk, rarely involve mucosa	Electrocardiographic conduction defects, ocular hypertelorism, pulmonary stenosis, abnormal genitalia, retardation of growth, and sensorineural deafness
PTEN hamartomatous syndrome Ruvalcaba-Myhre-Smith or Bannayan-Zonana syndrome (BRRS), and Cowden disease (CD)	Autosomal dominant	PTEN (10q23.31)	Lentiginosis plus	BRRS-delayed motor development, macrocephaly, lipomatosis, hamartomas CD-gingival papillomas, acral keratoses. Hamartomas, neoplasm-breast cancer, follicular thyroid cancer, and endometrial carcinoma
Centerofacial neurodysraphic lentiginosis	Autosomal dominant/ sporadic	Unknown	Lentiginosis involving malar area of cheek and nose predominantly and trunk	Mental retardation, central nervous system and endocrine abnormalities

Freckles are common during childhood, and primarily occur on sun exposed areas. Among genetic factors the melanocortin 1 receptor gene (MCR1) is major freckle gene which may play role in induction of phaeomelanogenesis. Clinically they present as round to oval brown pigmented macules with jagged margin. They lighten or disappear on avoidance of UV light exposure. Although they are considered risk factor for melanoma, usually they have benign course and fade with age. Histopathology shows basal layer hyperpigmentation without increase in melanocyte number. It is associated with neurofibromatosis type 1 where freckling is present in unexposed areas like axilla and palms.

Junctional nevus is common acquired melanocytic nevus which presents as a uniformly pigmented brown macule with diameter of 2–10 mm and often difficult to differentiate from lentigo on clinical grounds. Histopathology shows discrete nests of melanocytes/nevus cells at DEJ while in lentigo melanocytes do not form nests.

Seborrhoeic keratoses presents as sharply defined, light brown flat macule with velvety surface that gradually increase in size and thickness and develops into verrucous plaque to give stuck on skin appearance. Sometimes lesions may have greasy scale with smooth surface. It rarely occurs under age of 20 years. It involves covered as well as uncovered sites. Rarely, eruptive seborrhoeic keratoses are sign of internal malignancy most commonly gastric adenocarcinoma and this is known as the sign of Leser-Trélat.

Lentigo maligna also known as Hutchinson melanotic freckle is early form of melanoma. At early stage it presents as slowly growing light brown to dark brown or red-pink colored patch which may resemble freckle and lentigines sometimes. With time it becomes distinctive and atypical which can be identified by ABCDE rule of melanoma. Typical lesions of lentigo maligna characterized by variably pigmented light brown to dark brown or pink red colored irregular shaped patch with smooth surface. Lentigines and lentigo maligna can be differentiate by dermoscopy.

Lentigo simplex usually doesn't require any active treatment. Photoprotection may reduce number of new lesions. For cosmetic concern depigmenting agents, chemical peels, Q-switch Nd:Yag laser can be used with variable success.

Key Points
- Lentigo simplex is most common type of lentigo and usually starts in early childhood over photoexposed areas.
- Histopathology shows increased pigmentation of basal layer with slight increase in number of normal melanocytes.
- Avoidance of sun-exposure doesn't affect its course.

Diagnostic Pearls
- Clinical presentation in form of onset in early childhood and lesions are multiple, light brown to dark brown uniformly pigmented round to oval macules with irregular margins.
- Distribution involving predominantly photo-exposed sites with no history of disappearance on avoiding sun-exposure.
- Absence of systemic involvement

References

1. Praetorius C, Sturm RA, Steingrimsson E. Sun-induced freckling: ephelides and solar lentigines. Pigment Cell Melanoma Res. 2014;27(3):339–50.
2. Lallas A, Argenziano G, Moscarella E, Longo C, Simonetti V, Zalaudek I. Diagnosis and management of facial pigmented macules. Clin Dermatol. 2014;32(1):94–100.
3. Lodish MB, Stratakis CA. The differential diagnosis of familial lentiginosis syndromes. Familial Cancer. 2011;10(3):481–90.

Chapter 4
A 6 Years Old Male with Multiple Black Spots on Face

P. C. Das

A 6 years old male presented with the complaints of multiple black spots on the lips, perinasal and perioral areas since the early childhood. Personal history was remarkable for multiple episodes of abdominal colic and a few occurrences of rectal bleeding. There was history of having similar lesions in his sibling without any systemic complaint. On examination, gums, buccal mucosa, tongue and the hard palate were remarkable for multiple, discrete, brown to black pigmented macules (Figs. 4.1 and 4.2). Similar pigmented macules were present over the dorsum of fingers and toes and over the palms and soles (Fig. 4.3). Some nails had developed dark linear bands (melanonychia). The patient admits that all the spots except those over the lips were fading. Systemic examination was non-contributory. Based upon the above history and examination findings, what is the diagnosis?

1. LEOPARD syndrome
2. Peutz-Jegher's syndrome
3. Addison's disease
4. Laughier-Hunziker syndrome

P. C. Das (✉)
Apoorva Skin Centre, Katihar, India

© Springer Nature Switzerland AG 2020
S. Kothiwala et al. (eds.), *Clinical Cases in Disorders of Melanocytes*, Clinical Cases in Dermatology,
https://doi.org/10.1007/978-3-030-22757-9_4

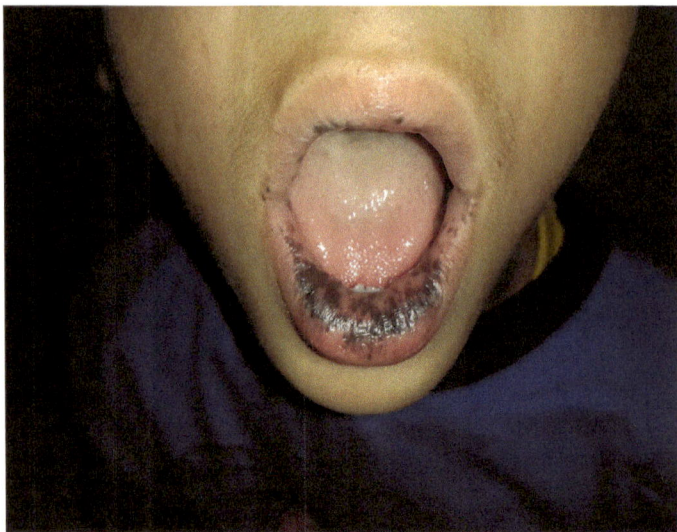

Figure 4.1 Young boy having dark brown coloured discrete and coalescing macule over lips. (Courtesy: Dr. Kanyarani Vashishth)

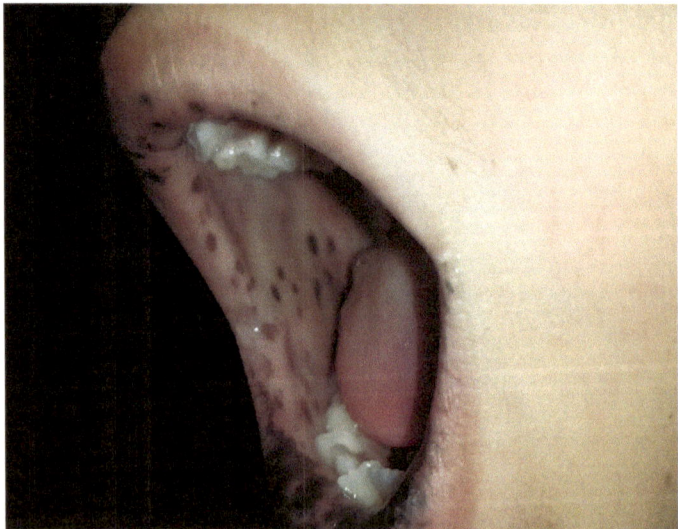

Figure 4.2 Pigmented macules on buccal mucosa. (Courtesy: Dr. Kanyarani Vashishth)

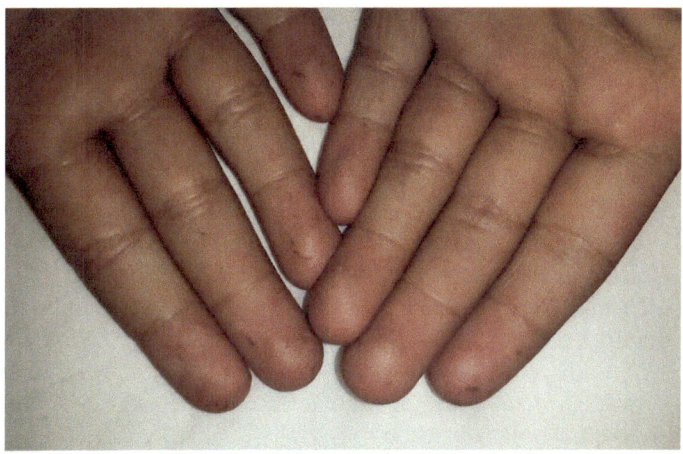

FIGURE 4.3 Pigmented macules of Peutz-Jegher's syndrome on palms. (Courtesy: Dr. Kanyarani Vashishth)

Diagnosis

- Peutz-Jegher's syndrome

Discussion

Peutz-Jegher's syndrome (PJS), also known as periorificial lentiginosis is a familial lentiginosis syndrome with autosomal dominant inheritance without any sex and racial preponderance. The condition develops due to mutation of a serine/threonine kinase 11gene (LKB1/STK11), located on chromosome 19p13 [1] and is characterised by mucocutaneous pigmentation, gastrointestinal polyps and increased risk of malignancies.

At birth or infancy onwards, dark brown-blue to brown-black pigmented macules of 2–4 mm size develop over lips, gums, buccal mucosa, hard palate, perioral, perinasal, periorbital, perianal skin, palms, soles, dorsum of finger and toes. Additionally, nails may show melanonychia. Except for mucosal lesions, these pigmented macules tend to fade away with time and by adulthood. Localization of pigmented macules in the oral mucosa is characteristic and very suggestive of Peutz-Jegher's syndrome. The diagnostic criteria put forward by World Health Organization (WHO) allows diagnosis of PJS if characteristic mucocutaneous pigmentation is present in a person with a family history of PJS.

Another hallmark of the disease is multiple benign polyps of the gastrointestinal tract. The common sites of affection are small intestine (64% in order of jejunum, ileum and duodenum), colon (63%), stomach (49%) and rectum (32%). The symptoms related to gastrointestinal polyposis are anaemia, vomiting, rectal bleeding, haematemesis, melaena, repeated abdominal colic, obstruction (usually of small intestine) and/or intussusception, infarction and extrusion of polyp. Symptomatic polyps usually present for the first time in adolescence and early adulthood; up to one-third of patients experience polyp-related symptoms by 10 years of age. Gastric outlet obstruction may present as early as in the neonatal period. Abdominal pain due to polyps causing subtotal obstruction increases in frequency and in intensity with age. Affected patients may develop extraintestinal polyps too; common manifestations include nasal polyps, gall bladder polyps, ureteric polyps, and respiratory tract polyps. These extraintestinal polyps too contribute to morbidity in patients with PJS [2].

The most feared complication is increased risk of malignancies both intestinal and extraintestinal. In general, risk of developing malignancy increases with age and is greater in females than in males. The most commonly reported include colon (39%), small intestine (13%), pancreatic (11–36%), stomach (29%), breast (45–50%), ovary (18–21%), and uterus (9%) cancers. Testicular carcinoma, lung carcinoma and thyroid carcinoma also have been reported [3]. Periodic follow up with endoscopy, colonoscopy, barium follow-through, biopsy and pelvic examination is required.

Diagnostic criteria based on the National Comprehensive Cancer Network (NCCN) 2018 guidelines includes presence of two or more of the following features: at least two biopsy proven Peutz-Jegher's-type hamartomatous polyps of the gastrointestinal (GI) tract; mucocutaneous hyperpigmentation affecting the eyes, nose, mouth/lips, fingers, or genitals; and a family history of Peutz-Jegher's syndrome [4].

Common clinical differential diagnoses include Laughier Hunziker syndrome, LEOPARD syndrome, Addison's disease and Bannayan-Riley-Ruvalcaba syndrome, as summarized in Table 4.1 [5].

For surveillance, genetic testing for mutations in the STK11 (LKB1) gene and thorough evaluation for early detection of malignancy is recommended [6]. Details family history of cancers and premalignant gastrointestinal conditions with the age of diagnosis, especially in first- and second-degree relatives,

TABLE 4.1 Summary of differential diagnosis of Peutz-Jegher's syndrome

Disease	Mucocutaneous features	Systemic features
LEOPARD syndrome	Lentigens distributed over neck, upper trunk, scalp, genitalia, palms and soles. Mucosa is spared	ECG abnormalities, ocular hypertelorism, pulmonary stenosis, abnormalities of genitalia, growth retardation and deafness
Addison's disease	diffuse hyperpigmentation of skin, darkening of elbows, creases of hands, freckles and bluish black macules on the mucous membranes	fatigability, weakness, anorexia, nausea, vomiting, weight loss and hypotension
Laugier Hunziker syndrome	Melanotic macules of oral cavity, longitudinal melanonychia	None
Bannayan-Riley-Ruvalcaba Syndrome	Pigmented macules of the glans penis	Macrocephaly, hamartomatous intestinal polyposis, lipomas

should be documented. This helps in determining the risk of a familial predisposition to cancer, and type and onset of cancer. Thus, surveillance can be tailor made for patients with PJS. Laboratory studies include complete blood cell count, iron studies, fecal occult blood, carcinoembryonic antigen (CEA), cancer antigen (CA)–19-9 and CA-125. Periodic colonoscopy, upper gastrointestinal endoscopy, Magnetic resonance imaging or ultrasound of the pancreas, chest X-ray, mammography and pelvic examination with ultrasound in women, and testicular examination in men are recommended for cancer screening [7].

Epidemiological studies and NCCN recommends screening for breast cancer at about age 25 years, Colon or stomach cancer in the late teens, small intestinal cancer at about age 8–10 years, pancreatic cancer at about age 30–35 years, ovarian/cervical/uterine cancer at about age 18–20 years and testicular (sex cord/Sertoli cell tumors) at about age 10 years in absence of family history of cancers. If there is any specific family history of cancer or suspicious symptoms, screening should be initiated earlier.

Peutz-Jegher's syndrome can be diagnosed early by detailed clinical examination, genetic testing in suspected individuals, screening for intestinal cancers and extraintestinal cancers. Genetic counselling, imaging studies and surgical treatment are part of management strategy for PJS [8]. Although mucocutaneous lesions fade away with age, sometimes laser treatment may be required for persistent skin lesions of cosmetic concern. Periodic endoscopic removal of all small intestinal polyps (at least polyps of more than 5 mm size) has a preventive role in polyp-related complications (discussed earlier) and helps avoid emergency laparotomy. Multidisciplinary approach with prevention and treatment of polyp-related complications, and surveillance for and treatment of various intestinal and extraintestinal malignancies form the cornerstone of management of patients with PJS.

Key Points

• Peutz-Jeghers syndrome is familial lentiginosis syndrome which is characterized by lentiginosis, hamartomatous GI polyps and neoplasm.

• It is autosomal dominant disorder with STK11/LKB1 mutation, although the type or site of STK11/LKB1 mutation do not significantly influence cancer risk.

• Cutaneous lesions are dark brown-blue pigmented lentigens at periorificial sites, lip, buccal mucosa, palate which develop in early childhood and tend to fade in late adulthood that may contribute to the difficulty in diagnosis.

• Genetic testing, counselling and screening for malignancy are the major parts of management.

References

1. McGarrity TJ, Amos C. Peutz-Jeghers syndrome: clinicopathology and molecular alterations. Cell Mol Life Sci. 2006;63(18):2135–44.

2. Zbuk KM, Eng C. Hamartomatous polyposis syndromes. Nat Clin Pract Gastroenterol Hepatol. 2007;4(9):492–502.

3. Hearle N, Schumacher V, Menko FH, Olschwang S, Boardman LA, Gille JJ, Keller JJ, Westerman AM, Scott RJ, Lim W, Trimbath JD, Giardiello FM, Gruber SB, Offerhaus GJ, de Rooij FW, Wilson JH, Hansmann A, Möslein G, Royer-Pokora B, Vogel T, Phillips RK, Spigelman AD, Houlston RS. Frequency and spectrum of cancers in the Peutz-Jeghers syndrome. Clin Cancer Res. 2006;12(10):3209–15.

4. The National Comprehensive Cancer Network. Clinical practice guidelines in oncology. Genetic/familial high-risk assessment: colorectal. Vol. 1. 2018. https://www.nccn.org/professionals/physician_gls/default.aspx#genetics_colon. Accessed 10 Oct 2018.

5. Lodish MB, Stratakis CA. The differential diagnosis of familial lentiginosis syndromes. Familial Cancer. 2011;10(3):481–90.

6. Van Lier MG, Wagner A, Mathus-Vliegen EM, Kuipers EJ, Steyerberg EW, van Leerdam ME. High cancer risk in Peutz-Jeghers syndrome: a systematic review and surveillance recommendations. Am J Gastroenterol. 2010;105(6):1258–64.

7. Kopacova M, Tacheci I, Rejchrt S, Bures J. Peutz-Jeghers syndrome: diagnostic and therapeutic approach. World J Gastroenterol. 2009;15(43):5397–408.
8. Beggs AD, Latchford AR, Vasen HF, Moslein G, Alonso A, Aretz S, Bertario L, Blanco I, Bülow S, Burn J, Capella G, Colas C, Friedl W, Møller P, Hes FJ, Järvinen H, Mecklin JP, Nagengast FM, Parc Y, Phillips RK, Hyer W, Ponz de Leon M, Renkonen-Sinisalo L, Sampson JR, Stormorken A, Tejpar S, Thomas HJ, Wijnen JT, Clark SK, Hodgson SV. Peutz-Jeghers syndrome: a systematic review and recommendations for management. Gut. 2010;59(7):975–86.

Chapter 5
20 Years Old Male with Multiple Hyperpigmented Macules on Trunk

Pawan Kumar

A 20 year old male presented with multiple hyperpigmented macule over trunk. He noticed it within first year of life after that it gradually increased in size in proportion to development. They are asymptomatic. There was no history of any other systemic complain. On examination he had five to six dark brown pigmented round to oval shaped sharply demarcated patch over right side of trunk (Fig. 5.1). Two macules were 3–4 cm in size while others were smaller. The lesions were uniformly hyperpigmented. Underlying soft tissue and appendages were normal. No other skin lesions were present. Based on this clinical information what is your diagnosis?

(a) Becker's Nevus
(b) Café-au-lait macule
(c) Congenital melanocytic nevus
(d) Nevus spilus

Diagnosis

- Café-au-lait macule

P. Kumar (✉)
Kempegowda Institute of Medical Sciences, Bengaluru, India

© Springer Nature Switzerland AG 2020   39
S. Kothiwala et al. (eds.), *Clinical Cases in Disorders of Melanocytes*, Clinical Cases in Dermatology,
https://doi.org/10.1007/978-3-030-22757-9_5

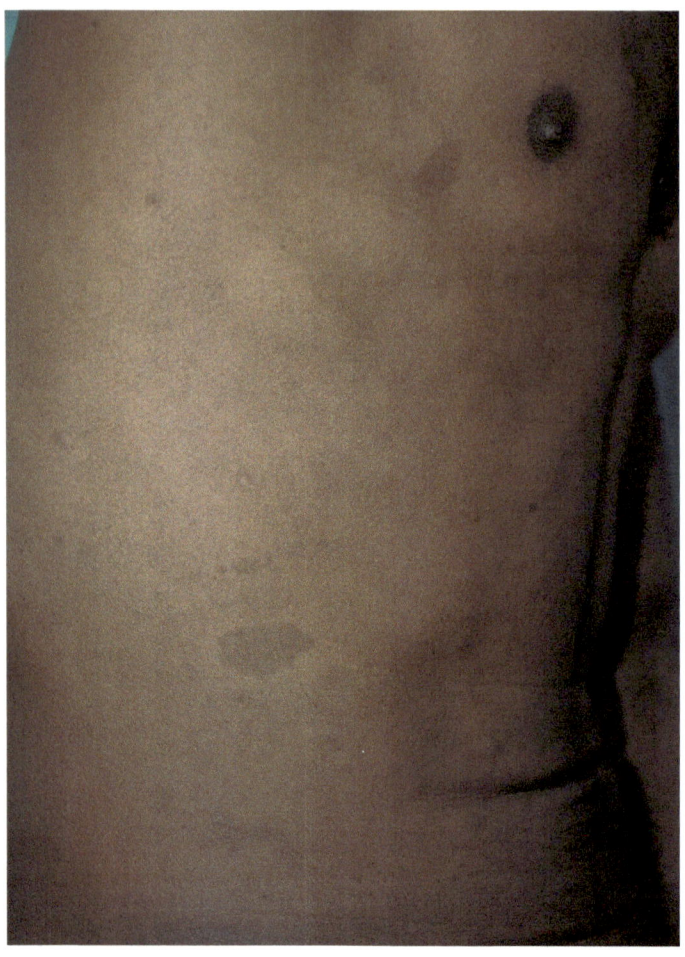

FIGURE 5.1 Five to six uniformly pigmented macules of variable size on trunk

Discussion

Café au lait macules (CALM) are localized epidermal mela-nocytic flat lesions, named after their typical coffee-and-milk hue. These are caused by an increase in melanin content, often with the presence of giant melanosomes. Café au lait macules (CALMS) are commonly noticed in childhood. In neonates, solitary CALMs may occurs in 0.3% of caucasians and 18% of African-Americans while in childhood it occurs in 13% of whites and 27% of blacks. At birth, a single CALM is observed in 5% of Caucasians. Three or more spots are observed in 2% of the population [1]. They often represent benign birthmarks but, however, they may also be markers of some systemic diseases.

Café-au-lait macules are round or oval shaped light to dark brown in colored macule with well demarcated smooth or irregular border. The pigment is evenly distributed. They can occur anywhere over the body, but individual lesions are more prevalent on unexposed skin. They are of varying sizes ranging from 2 mm to 20 cm, but usually under 2 cm in diameter [2]. There are two main types of CALMs. The most common type has fairly regular and clearly demarcated margins ("coast of California"). It is usually solitary/multiple and smaller in size. The second type is less frequent type of CALM that has a much more irregular margin ("coast of Maine"), and is usually larger and solitary. The distribution and configuration of café-au-lait macules can be a clue to an underlying syndrome.

CALMs may occur as isolated findings, or may be associated with minor and/or major congenital anomalies, as part of many syndromes. Multiple café-au-lait spots were observed in cancer predisposing syndromes (Table 5.1) like neurofibromatosis 1, neurofibromatosis 2, tuberous sclerosis, McCune-Albright syndrome, Fanconi anemia, LEOPARD syndrome, epidermal nevus syndrome, Bloom syndrome, ataxia-telangiectasia, and Silver–Russell syndrome [3]. More recently, café-au-lait spot were observed in 60% of carriers of biallelic mutations in mismatch repair (MMR) genes, characteristic of constitutional mismatch repair deficiency syndrome (CMMRDS) [4].

CALMs are typically observed in neurofibromatosis 1 (NF1), an autosomal dominant condition characterized by the presence of multiple neurofibromas, as well as other non-tumoral manifestations, like multiple CALMs, which are present in almost all adult patients with this disease, the

TABLE 5.1 Diseases associated with café-au-lait spots

Disorder	Other skin findings	Systemic involvement
Neurofibromatosis	Axillary freckling, neurofibromas	Sphenoid dysplasia, Lisch nodules (iris) Optic path glioma, neurologic involvement
McCune Albright syndrome	Few large café-au-lait spots	Polyostotic fibrous dysplasia, Hyperfunctioning hormonal disorders
Watson syndrome	Axillary freckling, neurofibromas	Pulmonary stenosis, mental retardation, short stature, relative macrocephaly, Lisch nodules on the iris
Silver–Russell dwarfism	Hypohidrosis in infancy	Small stature, skeletal asymmetry, clinodactyly of fifth finger, triangular face with prominent forehead
Ataxia-telangiectasia	Telangiectasia in bulbar conjunctivae and on face, sclerodermatous changes	Growth retardation, ataxia, mental retardation, lymphopenia, IgA, IgE, lymphoid tissue, respiratory infections
Tuberous sclerosis	Hypopigmented macules, shagreen patch, adenoma sebaceum, subungual fibromas	Central nervous system, kidneys, heart, lungs
Turner syndrome	Loose skin, especially around the neck, lymphedema in infancy, hemangiomas	Small stature, gonadal dysgenesis, skeletal anomalies, renal anomalies, cardiac defects

TABLE 5.1 (continued)

Disorder	Other skin findings	Systemic involvement
Bloom syndrome	Telangiectatic erythema of cheeks, photosensitivity, ichthyosis	Short stature, malar hypoplasia, risk of malignancy, immunodeficiency, distinctive narrow facies, high-pitched voice, hypogonadism and/or infertility
Multiple lentigines (LEOPARD syndrome)	Lentigines, axillary freckling	Electrocardiogram abnormalities, ocular hypertelorism, pulmonic stenosis, genital abnormalities, growth retardation, sensorineural deafness
Westerhof syndrome	Hypopigmented macules	Growth and mental retardation

CALMS of neurofibromatosis type-1, tends to have smooth margins that is likened to the coast of California.

McCune Albright syndrome is classically determined by a triad of CALMs, polyostotic fibrous dysplasia, and endocrine dysfunction. The café au lait spots in Albright syndrome has a predilection for the posterior aspect of neck, thorax, sacrum, and buttocks. They have a tendency to remain unilateral and to cover large anatomic regions. They are characteristic of irregular borders with jagged or serrated edges, resembling the coast of Maine in outline.

It is mainly a clinical diagnosis. A Wood lamp may improve the ability to visualize faint CALMs at early age. Skin biopsy reveals increased numbers of melanocytes and increased melanin in melanocytes and keratinocytes. Giant pigment granules have been identified in café-au-lait spots of neurofibromatosis. The presence of multiple cafe au lait macules should prompt a search for features suggestive of an underlying genetic disorder.

Becker naevus develops during puberty and presents as a large unilateral brown patch that break up into smaller macules at periphery. It develops commonly over upper back or chest but others sites like thighs, arm can also be involved. After puberty it often becomes darker and quite hairy, a feature also called hypertrichosis. Occasionally acne may develop in the naevus. Smooth muscle hamartoma and under development of underlying structures may also occur.

Congenital melanocytic naevi present at birth or within the first few months of life. It presents as solitary brown to black, round or oval-shaped pigmented patches with geographic borders. They may have increased hair growth (hypertrichosis). The surface may be slightly rough or bumpy with age.

Nevus spilus presents as tan or light brown colored patch at birth or soon after with darker brown macules or papules appearing within the lesion with age.

CALMs as such don't require any medical care and best advice is always counselling and reassurance but for some CALMs may be cosmetically troubling to patients. Anecdotal reports and case series suggest that laser therapy yields inconsistent results. Recently Q-switched 1064-nm Nd:YAG laser achieved good to excellent clearance in 74.4% of patients. Other lasers represented include the copper vapor laser, frequency-doubled Q-switched Nd:YAG, Q-switched ruby laser, Q-switched alexandrite laser, erbium-doped YAG, and pulsed-dye laser. Irregularly bordered coast of Maine lesions were far more likely to achieve good or excellent clearance than smooth-bordered coast of California lesions [5]. Risks for laser surgery include transient/permanent hyperpigmentation, hypopigmentation, and scarring. Treatment of underlying syndromes may be complex and require multidisciplinary care.

Key Points
- A café-au-lait macule is a common birthmark, presenting as a hyperpigmented skin patch with a sharp border and diameter of >0.5 cm.

- Isolated CALMs are invariably solitary and multiple CALMs are associated with several genetic syndromes.
- CALMs of NF-1 have smooth border while CALMs of McCune Albright syndrome have irregular order.

References

1. Cohen JB, Janniger CK, Schwartz RA. Café au lait spots. Paediatr Dermatol. 2000;66:22–4.
2. Tekin M, Bodurtha JN, Riccardi VM. Café au lait spots: the pediatrician's perspective. Pediatr Rev. 2001;22:82–90.
3. Shah KN. The diagnostic and clinical significance of café-au-lait macules. Pediatr Clin North Am. 2010;57:1131–53.
4. Wimmer K, Kratz CP, Vasen HF, Caron O, Colas C, Entz-Werle N, et al. Diagnostic criteria for constitutional mismatch repair deficiency syndrome: suggestions of the European consortium 'care for CMMRD' (C4CMMRD). J Med Genet. 2014;5:355–65.
5. Belkin DA, Neckman JP, Jeon H, Friedman P, Geronemus RG. Response to laser treatment of Café au lait macules based on morphologic features. JAMA Dermatol. 2017;153(11):1158–61.

Chapter 6
A 36 Year Old Woman with Hyperpigmented Macules on Face

Ashi and Sunil Kumar Kothiwala

A 36 year old woman presented with brownish patches bilaterally over malar area of her face, along forehead and nasal bridge. The lesions gradually increased in size and pigmentation over 3 years. Patient notices darkening of these patches on prolonged sun exposure especially in summer. The lady is a school teacher by profession. She applies sunscreen with SPF 25 once daily before going out in the sun. Apart from this she does not apply any other cosmetic products on her face. Her menstrual cycle is normal and general condition is good. She is married with one child 8 years old. She does not give history of similar lesions in past.

On examination, there were well demarcated multiple discrete to coalescing dark brown to light brown pigmented macules over cheeks, forehead, nose, chin and upper lip. Lesions were smooth surfaced with irregular margin, variable shape and non-uniform pigment intensity (Fig. 6.1). The skin on other parts of her face and neck are normal.

Based on the case description and the photograph, what is your diagnosis?

Ashi (✉)
Dermatologist, Sadar Hospital, Supaul, Bihar, India

S. K. Kothiwala
SkinEva Clinic, Jaipur, India

© Springer Nature Switzerland AG 2020   47
S. Kothiwala et al. (eds.), *Clinical Cases in Disorders of Melanocytes*, Clinical Cases in Dermatology,
https://doi.org/10.1007/978-3-030-22757-9_6

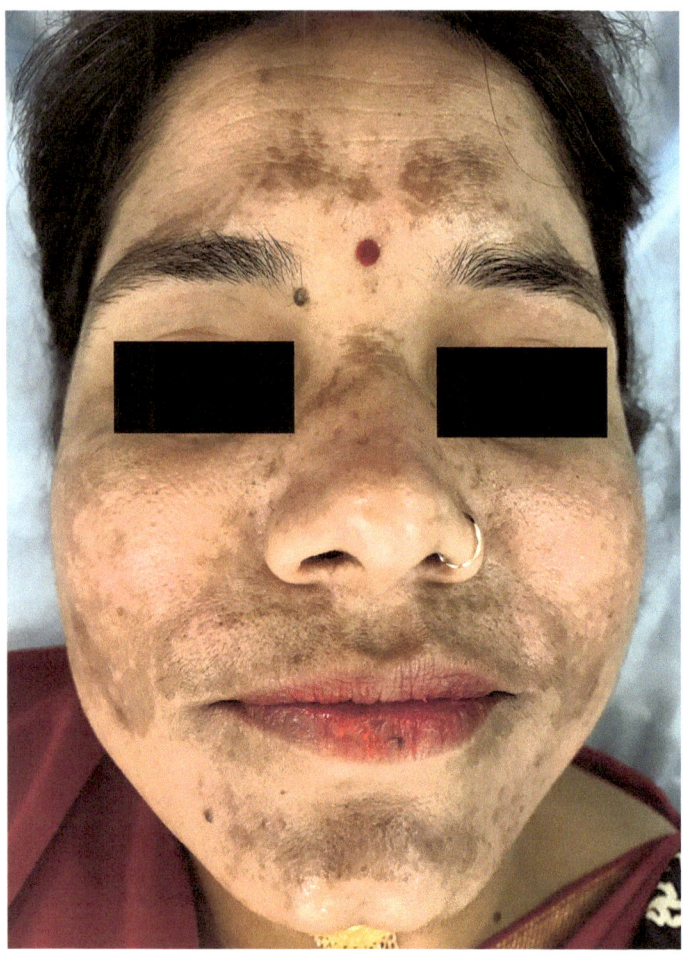

FIGURE 6.1 Multiple brown colored macules with irregular margin involving cheeks, nose, forehead, upper lip and chin

1. Post-inflammatory hyperpigmentation
2. Riehl's melanosis
3. Melasma
4. Exogenous ochronosis

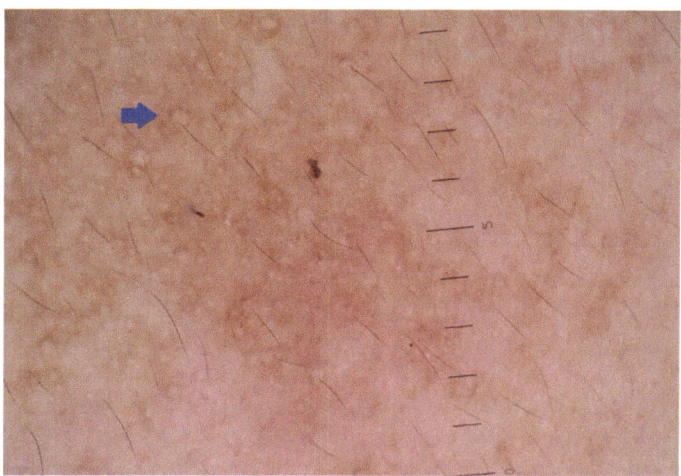

FIGURE 6.2 Dermoscopy showed pseudoreticular pattern of brown pigment; sparing of perifollicular area (blue arrow) (Courtesy: Dr. Sekhar Neema)

Woods lamp examination showed increased visibility of borders of macules at places with both enhancing and non-enhancing areas in lesion. Dermoscopy showed pseudoreticular network of brown pigment with sparing of perifollicular areas (Fig. 6.2).

Diagnosis

• Melasma

Discussion

Melasma is one of the most common chronic acquired pigmentary disorders. It is characterized by hyperpigmented macules present symmetrically mainly on the sun exposed areas of facc. Sun-cxposure and hormones are major triggering factors. Several clinical patterns of melasma including facial and extra-facial types have been described. Woods lamp examination helps in identifying epidermal, dermal or mixed types. There are several method of treatment including topical and oral medical treatment, chemical peels and lasers available for melasma.

The term chloasma (comes from Greek word *chloazein* meaning to be green) or the mask of pregnancy had been used in past, whereas the term melasma comes from the Greek *melas*, meaning brown. It occurs most commonly in Fitzpatrick skin phototype III and IV. Prevalence of melasma ranges from 1.5% in western countries [1] to as high as 40% Southeast Asian populations [2]. Melasma is much more common in women and occurs during reproductive years. It is present in 15–50% of pregnant patients.

The exact etiopathogenesis of melasma is not well understood; several factors have been reported. These risk factors are genetic predisposition, exposure to ultraviolet (UV) light, pregnancy, oral contraceptives and hormone replacement therapy [3]. Many studies have suggested higher incidence of melasma in family members indicating genetic predisposition a major risk factor. Sun exposure is a commonly reported aggravating factor because of UV-induced upregulation of melanocyte stimulating cytokines. Hormonal influence plays a role in development or exacerbation of melasma in some individuals. With pregnancy or oral contraceptive use onset or worsening of melasma has been noted in many patients but clinical evidence to date does not clearly associate serum hormone level to melasma. Other less common reported risk factors are cosmetic abuse, nutritional deficiency, thyroid disorders and phototoxic medications. Recent studies have suggested possibility of neural mechanism because of increased expression of nerve growth factor receptor (NGFR) in keratinocytes and more hypertrophic nerve fibers in superficial dermis of lesional skin compared to non-lesional skin. Increased expression of vascular endothelial growth factor (VEGF) by keratinocytes and more numerous large blood vessels in lesional skin indicate vascular component in pathogenesis of melasma. Histopathological studies have documented solar elastosis, basal layer vacuolar degeneration and basement membrane disruption, increased vascularity (evident by increased number, size and density of blood vessels), and increased mast cells in the lesional skin; the clinical and therapeutic implications of these findings are being explored. Considering increased vascularity of the lesional skin, tranexamic acid has been successfully tried in the treatment of melasma.

Patient with melasma show light brown to dark brown colored hyperpigmented macule or large patches with irregular border without any surface change. It may present with several distinct patterns:

(a) *Centrofacial pattern*—most common, involves cheeks, forehead, nose and upper lips.
(b) *Malar pattern*—cheek and nose
(c) *Mandibular pattern*—this may be form of poikiloderma of civatte and associated with chronic actinic damage.

Other rare described patterns are lateral cheek pattern and forearm pattern.

The diagnosis of melasma is usually straight forward and made clinically. Rarely it may require skin biopsy to differentiate from other pigmentary disorders. Histopathologically it is characterized by presence of melanin deposition in basal and suprabasal layers (epidermal melasma) or superficial and deep perivascular melanophages in the dermis (dermal melasma) with highly dendritic (branched) deeply pigmented melanocytes and some degree of solar elastosis. Dermoscopy is a more accurate tool used nowadays for the diagnosis and classification of melasma based on depth. Lesions of epidermal melasma show diffuse reticular pigmentation in various shades of brown with sparing of follicular openings. Dermal melasma shows diffuse dark brown to grayish pseudo-reticular pigmentation [4]. In addition, annular, honeycomb and arcuate structures can also be seen.

Reflectance confocal microscopy is a more advanced non-invasive tool that depicts changes in the skin and pigmentation upto papillary dermis thus providing images with resolution like that of histopathological examination [5]. It can be used for determining prognosis based on depth as well as monitoring response to therapy.

Other disorders that may be need to be differentiated from melasma are: postinflammatory hyperpigmentation, solar lentigines, freckles, drug-induced pigmentation, actinic lichen planus, lichen planus pigmentosus, facial acanthosis, frictional melanosis, nevus of Ota and naevus of Hori [6].

Post inflammatory hyperpigmentation (PIH) can occur at any age without any gender preference. It presents as asymptomatic hyperpigmented macules and patches ranging in color from light brown to bluish grey. There is history of preceding inflammatory event such as allergic reaction, drug and phototoxic reaction, infections, injury and inflammatory dermatoses [7]. Epidermal PIH usually occurs as a result of stimulation of melanocytes after inflammatory events like acne, pyoderma, atopic dermatitis, psoriasis, pityriasis rosea and insect bites and generally resolves with time in months. Dermal PIH develops when there is disruption of basal cell layer leading to melanin incontinence and capture by melanophages in the papillary dermis as with lupus erythematous and fixed drug reaction and it takes more time in resolution than epidermal.

Riehl's melanosis or pigmented contact dermatitis as the name suggests is postulated to be caused by frequent and repeated contact with small amounts of sensitizing allergens primarily in cosmetic and textile materials. It is an allergic contact dermatitis due to type IV hypersensitivity reaction. The mechanism involves damage to the basal layer of epidermis followed by pigmentary incontinence. It is more common in Mexican and Asian female.

Exogenous ochronosis is an uncommon and acquired condition which is limited to skin and is clinically and histologically similar to its endogenous counterpart alkaptonuria which is an inherited disorder with systemic effects. Exogenous ochronosis presents as asymptomatic bilaterally symmetrical speckled blue-black or gray-black macules, sometimes papules and nodules. It typically affects the malar areas, temples, lower cheeks, and neck. It most commonly results from the prolonged use of topical hydroquinones, though the use of phenol, quinine, resorcinol, picric acid, mercury, and oral anti-malarials has also been associated with this condition [8]. Many theories have been put forth to explain its pathogenesis. The most accepted theory states that the hyperpigmentation is due to local competitive inhibition of the enzyme homogentisic oxidase by hydroquinone. This in turn leads to local accumulation of homogentisic acid and its metabolic products that polymerizes to form typical ochronotic pigment in the papillary dermis. Wood's lamp examination and ultraviolet light photography are noninvasive techniques for differentiating melasma and EO but have not provided promising results as the two conditions can co-exist. Dermoscopy reveals dark brown globules and globular-like structures on a diffuse brown background [9]. Reflectance confocal microscopy shows the presence of hyporefractile oval-to-banana-shaped spaces in the dermis. The pathognomic gold-standard histopathological feature is the presence of the ochre-colored, banana-shaped fibers in the dermis. Homogenization and swelling of collagen bundles in the papillary and reticular dermis may also be seen [10].

Melasma is a relatively easy condition to diagnose but a difficult one to treat. Resistant cases and recurrences of melasma occur often more so if strict avoidance of sunlight is not undertaken. Several treatment options are available for melasma including topical formulations, chemical peels, and lasers [11]. Use of a broad-spectrum topical sunscreen that protects against both UVA and visible light is recommended.

Depigmenting agent hydroquinone, retinoids alone or in combination, azelaic acid, kojic acid, ascorbic acid and arbutin are major topical formulation effective in melasma. Oral tranexamic acid is a plasmin inhibitor and have been shown to be efficacious in melasma [12]. Among chemical peels glycolic acid peels are most efficacious and other peels like Jessner solution (composed of salicylic acid, lactic acid, and resorcinol) and trichloroacetic acid have been used in melasma. Intense pulse light has shown moderately satisfying results in topical therapy refractory melasma. Q-switched Nd-YAG has the added advantage of being effective in the dermal aspect of melasma because of its deeper penetration [13]. The pulse dye laser (PDL) is an emerging modality that targets the vascular component in melasma lesions. It decreases melanocyte stimulation and probably even the subsequent relapses. Fractional laser therapy appears to be most promising laser or light treatment for melasma but should be done with precautions to avoid post procedure hyperpigmentation. Although results are not consistent with any single or combination of treatment modalities, selection of therapy depends on patient's disease severity and impact on quality of life while keeping in mind benefits and risks of various treatments.

Key Points

- Melasma an acquired chronic disorder of melanogenesis that presents with brown to gray black hyperpigmented macules or patches with irregular border in almost always symmetrical distribution. Increased expression of vascular and neural growth factors also play a role in pathogenesis of melasma.
- Sun exposure and hormonal factors are most studied exacerbating factors which make photoprotection and avoidance of oral contraceptives major part of management.
- Dermal melasma is more difficult to treat with topical depigmenting agents.
- Topical formulations are the basic key of the treatment, chemical peels, lights and laser therapy may be considered with precautions in resistant cases.

References

1. Werlinger KD, Guevara IL, González CM, Rincón ET, Caetano R, Haley RW, et al. Prevalence of self-diagnosed melasma among premenopausal Latino women in Dallas and Fort Worth, Tex. Arch Dermatol. 2007;143:424–5.
2. Sivayathorn A. Melasma in orientals. Clin Drug Invest. 1995;10(Suppl 2):34–40.
3. Sheth VM, Pandya AG. Melasma: a comprehensive update: part I. J Am Acad Dermatol. 2011;65:689–97.
4. Sarkar R, Arora P, Garg VK, Sonthalia S, Gokhale N. Melasma update. Indian Dermatol Online J. 2014;5:426–35.
5. Kang HY, Bahadoran P, Suzuki I, Zugaj D, Khemis A, Passeron T, et al. In vivo reflectance confocal microscopy detects pigmentary changes in melasma at a cellular level resolution. Exp Dermatol. 2010;19:e228–33.
6. Handog EB, Macarayo MJ. Melasma and vitiligo in brown skin. New Delhi: Springer; 2017.
7. Kaufman BP, Aman T, Alexis AF. Postinflammatory hyperpigmentation: epidemiology, clinical presentation, pathogenesis and treatment. Am J Clin Dermatol. 2018;19(4):489–503.
8. Levin CY, Maibach H. Exogenous ochronosis. An update on clinical features, causative agents and treatment options. Am J Clin Dermatol. 2001;2:213–7.
9. Gil I, Segura S, Martínez-Escala E, Lloreta J, Puig S, Vélez M, et al. Dermoscopic and reflectance confocal microscopic features of exogenous ochronosis. Arch Dermatol. 2010;146:1021–5.
10. Tan SK. Exogenous ochronosis in ethnic Chinese Asians: a clinicopathological study, diagnosis and treatment. J Eur Acad Dermatol Venereol. 2011;25:842–50.
11. Ogbechie OA, Elbuluk N. Melasma: an up-to-date comprehensive review. Dermatol Ther. 2017;7:305–18.
12. Zhang L, Tan WQ, Fang QQ, Zhao WY, Zhao QM, Gao J, Wang XW. Tranexamic acid for adults with melasma: a systematic review and meta-analysis. Biomed Res Int. 2018;2018:1683414.
13. Trivedi MK, Yang FC, Cho BK. A review of laser and light therapy in melasma. Int J Womens Dermatol. 2017;3(1):11–20.

Chapter 7
A 24 Year Old Male with Hyperpigmented Macules in Face, Neck and Upper Extremities

Dipak Kumar Agarwalla

A 24 year male presented with multiple grey brown macules on face, neck and upper trunk since 6 months. It was insidious in onset and gradually progressive. It was not preceded by any erythema over the lesions and was asymptomatic. There was no history of any application of cosmetics. On examination patient had discrete as well as confluent slate grey coloured hyperpigmented macules with ill-defined border distributed over face, neck and upper limb (Fig. 7.1). The surface was smooth and non-scaly. Oral cavity, nails, palms and soles were not affected.

Based on the case description and figure, what is your diagnosis?

1. Lichen planus pigmentosus
2. Erythema dyschromicum perstans
3. Reihl's melanosis
4. Macular amyloidosis
5. Postinflammatory pigmentation

D. K. Agarwalla (✉)
Gauhati Medical College and Hospital, Guwahati, India

© Springer Nature Switzerland AG 2020
S. Kothiwala et al. (eds.), *Clinical Cases in Disorders of Melanocytes*, Clinical Cases in Dermatology,
https://doi.org/10.1007/978-3-030-22757-9_7

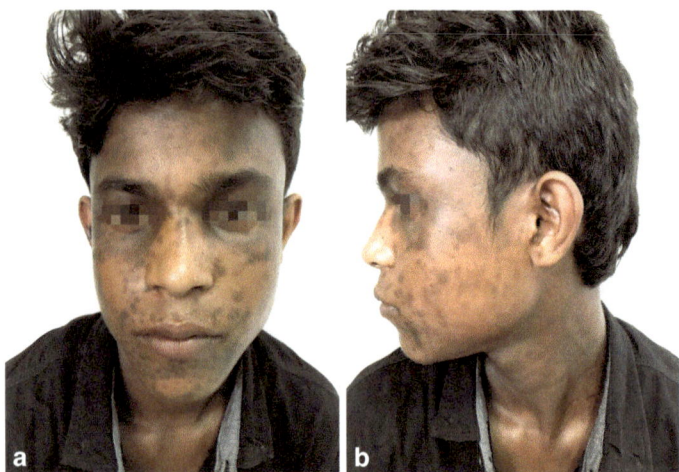

FIGURE 7.1   Blue-grey hyperpigmented macules on face (**a**) and neck (**b**) in a 24 year old male

Dermoscopy reveals grey to blue pigment dots forming a net like pattern with reticular pigment network (Fig. 7.2). Histopathology showed marked pigmentary incontinence, focal basal cell degeneration with minimal perivascular lymphocytic infiltrate in superficial dermis.

Diagnosis

- Lichen planus pigmentosus

Discussion

Lichen planus pigmentosus (LPP) is considered to be a rare variant of lichen planus (LP). It predominantly affects patients with darker skin phototypes III to IV and commonly observed in India, Latin America and Africa. The onset occurs between third to fifth decades of life. Most of studies have reported female preponderance. In India, LPP has been

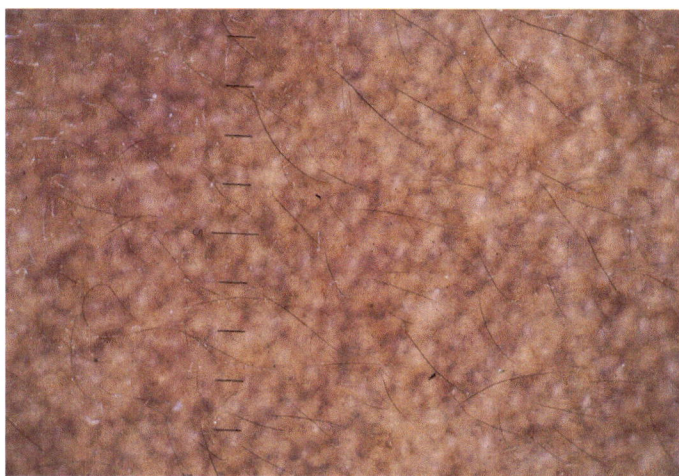

FIGURE 7.2 Grey to blue pigment dots which are bigger in size and forming a net like pattern and reticular pigment network in dermoscopy (Courtesy: Dr. Shekhar Neema)

linked with use of mustard oil containing photo-sensitizer (allyl-thiocyanate), amla oil, henna and hair dye. In Kuwait, association with hepatitis C virus infection has been reported. Sun exposure and hormonal factors have also been considered as exacerbating factors.

LPP similar to LP shows altered cellular immune response mediated by CD8+ T lymphocytes. LP has been considered an abortive variant of LP, in which a rapid inflammatory event destroys epidermal keratinocytes without compensatory keratinocyte proliferation followed by rapid regression of the inflammatory infiltrate. It results in intense pigmentary incontinence which remains for months to years.

Clinically it is characterized by a symmetrical distribution of slate grey to brown black, round to oval macules with poorly defined borders. Macules gradually enlarge and coalesce. The pigmentation may be diffuse, reticulate, blotchy or perifollicular. LPP mainly affects the face, neck, arm and upper trunk. On face, sun-exposed sites like temporal and preauricular areas are more affected. Rarely oral mucosa and scalp may get involved. Palms, soles and nails are not involved. LP lesions may rarely be associated with LPP. The lesions are usually asymptomatic. Mild itching may be present in 27–62% of patients which is marker of activity and progression of disease [1]. With time it resolves. Few patients may complain of burning sensation. Disease have chronic course with remission and relapses.

LPP inversus is the most important variant wherein the lesions are present in the flexors, intertriginous areas and other skin folds with sparing of sun-exposed sites. The lesions are distributed with longitudinal axis along the lines of cleavage [2]. It is more common in fair individuals and friction and tight clothing have been proposed as triggers. Other variants are LPP along Blaschko's lines (linear LPP), zosteriform LPP.

Histopathology of new lesions of LPP shows vacuolar degeneration of basal cell layer, band-like lichenoid or perivascular lymphocytic infiltrate in the papillary dermis, pigmentary incontinence and melanophages. Older lesions show marked pigmentary incontinence, melanophages with minimal vacuolar degeneration and slight perivascular inflammatory infiltrate. Direct immunofluorescence reveals globular deposition of IgM in the papillary dermis and dermal-epidermal junction, but it is positive in 7–16% of cases [1]. With Wood's light examination, there is no enhancement, because melanin is predominantly located in dermis. Dermoscopy of LPP shows brown homogenous areas that represent epidermal pigmentation and gray-brown or gray-blue dots and globules that represent pigmentary incontinence and melanophages in papillary demis. In early lesions gray dots grouped in a diffuse black pepper-like pattern but with time they converge to form reticular, linear and cobblestone patterns. White dots represent absence of pigmentation in follicular openings and skin creases [3].

Common differential diagnosis are erythema dyschromicum perstans (EDP), reihl's melanosis, macular amyloidosis, post inflammatory hyperpigmentation, melasma, fixed drug eruption, hori nevus and ochronosis.

EDP has remarkable clinical and histopathological similarities to LPP and differ slightly in color, border and distribution of lesions. EDP presents with ash coloured macules with slightly elevated erythematous margins. They are asymptomatic and later merge, losing the erythematous borders. The trunk, arms and neck can be involved with predilection for non-sun exposed areas. Pruritus is less common than LPP [4].

Reihl's melanosisis thought to be a pigmented contact dermatitis to allergens present in cosmetics or fragrances. It presents as patches of diffuse gray-brown pigmentation on forehead, scalp, face, and neck. Erythema, scaling or pruritus is occasionally present. Prior history of topical application and positive patch test identifying the allergen predicts the diagnosis.

Macular amyloidosis affects women more often than men. Macular dark brown pigmentation occurs commonly in interscapular space but can involve shins, thighs, arms, extremities, and face. The lesions consist of rippled or reticulated pigmentation which is typically pruritic.

Postinflammatory pigmentation has a history of preexisting inflammation and the pattern of pigmentation may predict the underlying condition. The lesions are usually ill-defined and may show areas with patchy hypopigmentation [5].

Management of LPP includes avoidance of trigging factors, topical and systemic medications and lasers. Topical agents have been tried with variable success in subsiding inflammation and decreasing pigmentation. It includes topical corticosteroids, tacrolimus, and skin lightening creams having hydroquinone and retinoids. Oral corticosteroids in pulsed or continuous doses with tapering, dapsone 100 mg, isotretinoin 0.3 mg/kg/day are systemic agents which have shown efficacy in stopping disease progression and reducing hyperpigmentation. Although it is not well known that continuation of systemic therapy for long to prevent relapses is appropriate or not. Q-switch Nd:Yag laser in conjunction with tacrolimus have shown low moderate efficacy.

Key Points

- LPP shares pathogenesis with LP by showing abnormal immune response mediated by CD8+ cells which results in damage to keratinocytes. Early lesions show vacuolar degeneration of basal layer with inflammatory infiltrate while older lesions show marked pigmentary incontinence.
- LPP is characterized by asymptomatic symmetrical slate grey to brown black macules with diffuse border involving the sun exposed areas especially face, neck and upper limbs.
- Dermoscopic features include absence of wickham striae, diffuse brown colour and pseudoreticular pigment network, slate gray to blue dots and globules, perifollicular and peri-eccrine gray to brown/gray blue pigment deposition.
- Treatment are not so effective with variable response to vitamin A, oral and topical steroids, tacrolimus, photoprotection and pigment laser.

References

1. Kanwar AJ, Dogra S, Handa S, Parsad D, Radotra BD. A study of 124 Indian patients with lichen planus pigmentosus. Clin Exp Dermatol. 2003;28(5):481–5.
2. Robles-Méndez JC, Rizo-Frías P, Herz-Ruelas ME, Pandya AG, OcampoCandiani J. Lichen planus pigmentosus and its variants: review and update. Int J Dermatol. 2018;57(5):505–14.
3. Güngör S, Topal IO, Göncü EK. Dermoscopic patterns in active and regressive lichen planus and lichen planus variants: a morphological study. Dermatol Pract Concept. 2015;5(2):45–53.
4. Ghosh A, Coondoo A. Lichen planus pigmentosus: the controversial consensus. Indian J Dermatol. 2016;61:482–6.
5. Mathews I, Thappa DM, Singh N, Gochhait D. Lichen planus pigmentosus: a short review. Pigment Int. 2016;3:5–10.

Chapter 8
A 25-Year Old Woman with Scaly Hypopigmented Lesions

Preeti Sharma

A 25-year-old female presented to our outpatient department complaining of multiple asymptomatic hypopigmented, mildly scaly lesions gradually increasing in number and size, present over upper trunk, neck and upper arms. Lesions appeared whitish and became prominent on wetting at the time of taking bath (Fig. 8.1). On clinical examination, there were well-defined hypopigmented macules of 4–5 mm in diameter at places coalescing to form irregular patches with furfuraceous scales present over anterior chest, upper back, proximal arms and neck. Some of the patches had wrinkled appearance. On performing scratch test with slide, accentuation of scaling was observed. Microscopic examination of potassium hydroxide (KOH) mounted skin scrapings demonstrated fungal spores and short, broad, branched hyphae (Fig. 8.2).

Based on the case description and photographs, what is your diagnosis?

1. Pityriasis rosea
2. Pityriasis versicolor
3. Pityriasis lichenoides chronica
4. Seborrheic Dermatitis

P. Sharma (✉)
All India Institute of Medical Sciences, Patna, India

© Springer Nature Switzerland AG 2020   63
S. Kothiwala et al. (eds.), *Clinical Cases in Disorders of Melanocytes*, Clinical Cases in Dermatology,
https://doi.org/10.1007/978-3-030-22757-9_8

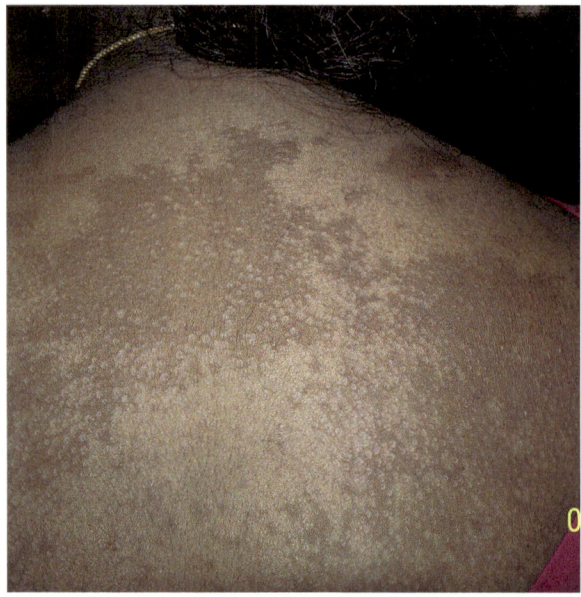

Figure 8.1 Multiple hypopigmented macules and patches with fine scales on upper back (Courtesy: Dr. Piyush Kumar)

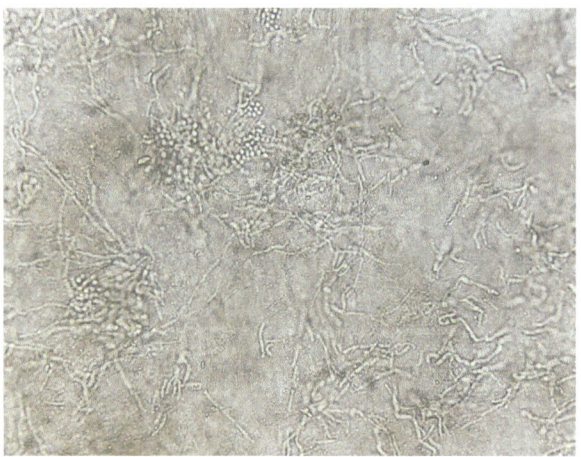

Figure 8.2 KOH mount showing thick-walled spherical yeast in clusters, with short fungal filaments (Courtesy: Dr. Piyush Kumar)

Diagnosis

- Pityriasis versicolor (Tinea versicolor)

Discussion

Pityriasis versicolor (PV), also known as tinea versicolor is a superficial, recurring fungal infection of the stratum corneum, characterized by scaly, dyspigmented irregular macules most often occurring on the trunk and extremities [1]. *Malassezia* yeast, a dimorphic fungus, is the causative organism whose mycelial form is mainly responsible for clinicopathologic changes [2]. Currently 12 species of this dimorphic fungus are known; commonly implicated ones are *M. furfur*, *M. sympodialis*, and *M. globosa* [3].

As mentioned earlier, PV may present with both hypopigmented and hyperpigmented macules and patches; sometimes, both types of lesions are noted in same patient. In general, dark-skinned population develops hypopigmented lesions, while hyperpigmented lesions are common in people with lighter skin color. The hypopigmentation in PV is caused by azelaic acid (a dicarboxylic acid produced by fungus) mediated inhibition of tyrosinase enzyme [4]. Malassezin, another metabolite from fungus, is implicated in causing apoptosis of melanocytes and may have a contributory role in causing hypopigmented lesions. On the other hand, hyperpigmentation is believed to be caused by abnormally large melanosomes [5], a thick stratum corneum [6], and a hyperemic inflammatory response [7, 8]. *Malassezia* spp. secrete other metabolites like pityriacitrin, pityrialactone, etc. which are responsible for fluorescence produced under wood's lamp.

Malassezia spp. is a common commensal, present over seborrheic areas of the body (head, scalp and central trunk) and usually does not cause disease. Various predisposing factors which results in transition of normal commensal form of this dimorphic fungus into pathogenic mycelia form are hot and humid environment, hyperhidrosis, immunosuppressed state, use of medications like systemic corticosteroids, oral contraceptives, and malnourished state [9]. Other than PV, *Malassezia* sp. is implicated in Pityrosporum folliculitis and Seborrheic dermatitis.

Clinical appearance of PV is characteristic enough to clinch the diagnosis and is characterized by scaly oval to round macules coalescing to form patches of pigmentary alteration ranging from almost white to pink to reddish brown with dust like scales and wrinkled surface present over upper trunk and extremities, with macules starting in perifollicular location (vide Fig. 8.1) and then coalescing. On scratching the lesions, extensive scaling is produced (Scratch sign or coup d'ongle sign). Wood's lamp examination helps in making the diagnosis and potassium hydroxide (KOH) examination is confirmatory. Biopsy is rarely required and periodic acid-Schiff (PAS) staining reveals oval budding yeast and branching hyphae which appears as 'banana and grapes' or 'spaghetti and meat balls'.

The common differential diagnoses include pityriasis lichenoides chronica, pityriasis rosea and seborrheic dermatitis. Pityriasis lichenoides chronica starts with erythematous scaly papules which leave hypopigmented macules on healing, and runs a longer course. Pityriasis rosea has a history of herald patch, followed by development of secondary lesions along the lines of cleavage in a Christmas tree pattern. The individual lesion is annular with collarette of scales. Seborrheic dermatitis is characterized by greasy loose or adherent scales, involvement of scalp, glabella, ala nasi, retroauricualr area, sternal area, midscapular area, and flexures. This itchy condition runs a chronic relapsing course.

PV is treated by topical and oral antifungals with some life style modifications (avoiding prolonged exposure to hot, humid environment if possible, changing wet under garments frequently, frequent baths etc.). Topical treatment can be divided into specific ones having fungistatic activity and non-specific ones. Topical antifungals bifonazole, clotrimazole, oxiconazole, and miconazole have direct fungistatic activity. Most commonly prescribed topical antifungals are ketoconazole shampoo and 1% terbinafine cream. Selenium sulphide (lotion, cream, or shampoo), and zinc pyrithione are other helpful agents.

Non-specific topical measures act by physically or chemically removing the superficial dead infected skin layers. Non-specific treatments include propylene glycol, and Whitfield's ointment [10, 11].

Among systemic antifungals, terbinafine is not effective in treatment of PV as it is not secreted in sweat and doesn't reach the required concentration in the stratum corneum. Ketoconazole, once the gold standard in treating PV, is no longer used because of its FDA Black Box warning of hepatotoxicity. Effective systemic agents include itraconazole, fluconazole and pramiconazole and are reserved for extensive/chronically recurring cases. The commonly used regimens are

- Fluconazole 400 mg single dose
- Itraconazole 200 mg daily for 5 days
- Pramiconazole 200 mg daily for 3 days

Patients are advised to remain in cooler environment to avoid sweating and take frequent baths atleast twice a day. Itraconazole 400 mg once a month can be added to prevent recurrences [12].

Key Points
- Pityriasis versicolor is a common superficial fungal infection of skin. It is particularly common among people who work/reside in hot, humid environment.
- Pityriasis versicolor clinically presents with well-defined hypopigmented oval to round macules over sebaceous rich areas. Presence of perifollicular lesions is a useful diagnostic clue.
- Diagnosis is mainly clinical and potassium hydroxide (KOH) mount is confirmatory.
- Treatment is mainly topical therapy and oral antifungals can be prescribed as second line therapy in resistant/extensive lesions.

References

1. Kallini JR, Riaz F, Khachemoune A. Tinea versicolor in dark-skinned individuals. Int J Dermatol. 2014;53(2):137–41.
2. Gupta AK, Bluhm R, Summerbell R. Pityriasis versicolor. J Eur Acad Dermatol Venereol. 2002;16:19–33.
3. Crespo-Erchiga V, Florencio VD. Malassezia yeasts and pityriasis versicolor. Curr Opin Infect Dis. 2006;19:139–47.
4. Mendez-Tovar LJ. Pathogenesis of dermatophytosis and tinea versicolor. Clin Dermatol. 2010;28(2):185–9.
5. Allen HB, Charles CR, Johnson BL. Hyperpigmented tinea versicolor. Arch Dermatol. 1976;112:1110–2.
6. Galadari I, el Komy M, Mousa A, Hashimoto K, Mehregan AH. Tinea versicolor: histologic and ultrastructural investigation of pigmentary changes. Int J Dermatol. 1992;31:253–6.
7. Dotz WI, Henrikson DM, Yu GS, Galey CI. Tinea versicolor: a light and electron microscopic study of hyperpigmented skin. J Am Acad Dermatol. 1985;12:37–44.
8. Papa CM, Kligman AM. The behavior of melanocytes in inflammation. J Invest Dermatol. 1965;45:465–73.
9. Sunenshine PJ, Schwartz RA, Janniger CK. Tinea versicolor. Int J Dermatol. 1998;37(9):648–55.
10. Gupta AK, Batra R, Bluhm R, Faergemann J. Pityriasis versicolor. Dermatol Clin. 2003;21:413–29.
11. Gupta AK, Kogan N, Batra R. Pityriasis versicolor: a review of pharmacological treatment options. Expert Opin Pharmacother. 2005;6:165–78.
12. Gupta AK, Lyons DC. Pityriasis versicolor: an update on pharmacological treatment options. Expert Opin Pharmacother. 2014;15(12):1707–13.

Chapter 9
A Lady with Facial Pigmentation

Dhiraj Kumar

A 36-year-old woman presented to department of dermatology with complaint of dark discoloration of face for last 2 years. She gave history of application of some cosmetic cream 2 months prior to the onset of presenting complaint. The discoloration started as a reddish patch, associated with burning sensation followed by hyperpigmentation. The nature of cream was not known to the patient. No history of pre-existing dermatosis or photosensitivity was noted. There were no other associated cutaneous and systemic co-morbidities.

On cutaneous examination, there was diffuse dark-brown to greyish-brown facial pigmentation, most pronounced on the lateral aspects of face and neck particularly concentrated on the forehead, and around the eyes (Fig. 9.1). Margins were irregular and surface was non-scaly. Oral mucosa and conjunctiva were spared. Rest of the dermatological and systemic examinations were unremarkable. Dermoscopy of the lesion showed small, discrete, brown to grey pigmented dots that do not form a net like pattern (Fig. 9.2).

D. Kumar (✉)
All India Institute of Medical Sciences, Patna, India

© Springer Nature Switzerland AG 2020
S. Kothiwala et al. (eds.), *Clinical Cases in Disorders of Melanocytes*, Clinical Cases in Dermatology,
https://doi.org/10.1007/978-3-030-22757-9_9

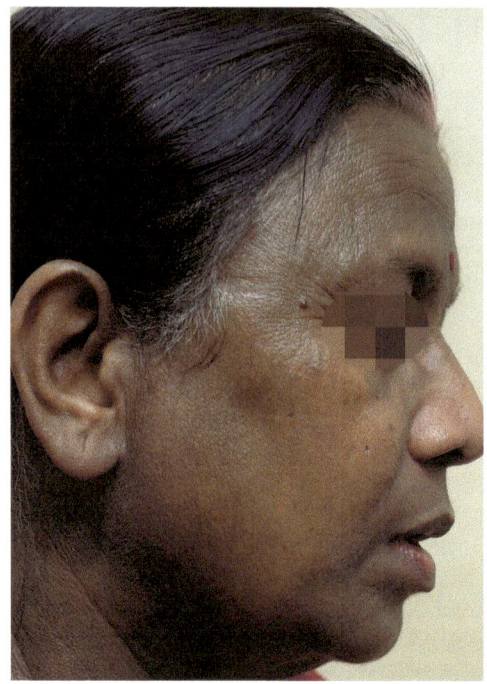

FIGURE 9.1 Hyperpigmented macules and patches on the forehead and sides of the face (Courtesy: Dr. Piyush Kumar)

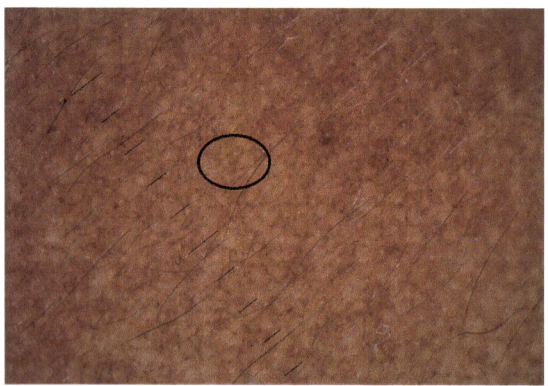

FIGURE 9.2 Dermoscopy showing small, discrete, brown to grey pigmented dots that do not form a net like pattern (Courtesy: Dr. Shekhar Neema)

Based on the history and clinical presentation, what is your diagnosis?

1. Melasma
2. Lichen planus pigmentosus (LPP)
3. Pigmented contact dermatitis (Riehl'smelanosis)
4. Exogenous ochronosis

Diagnosis

- Pigmented contact dermatitis (Riehl's melanosis)

Discussion

Pigmented contact dermatitis (PCD), also known as Riehl's melanosis, is a non-eczematous variant of contact dermatitis. In this condition, clinical picture is dominated by acquired hyperpigmentation with little or no signs of dermatitis [1]. Osmundsen, a Danish dermatologist had first used the term "pigmented contact dermatitis" to describe an epidemic of contact dermatitis in Copenhagen which had occurred due to the optical whitener (Tinopal CH 3566) used in washing powders [2]. The unique pattern of pigmentation as seen in PCD was first noted by Riehl during World War I, but Riehl could not establish the cause and attributed the pigmentation to nutritional deficiency in wartime conditions.

The exact mechanism by which these allergens induce pigmentation is unknown. Osmundsen considered it an idiosyncratic reaction. The allergen responsible for PCD may have a special affinity for melanin, inciting an inflammatory reaction first around the melanocytes and then around the cells incorporating melanin granules [3]. Nakayama et al. hypothesized that the concentrations of allergens in commercial preparations were too low to produce spongiotic dermatitis. Instead, they produced cytolytic type of type IV allergy mainly at the basal layer of the epidermis that resulted in pigmentary incontinence [4].

Commonly implicated allergens in the development of pigmented contact dermatitis are summarized in Table 9.1

TABLE 9.1 Common chemicals implicated in pigmented contact dermatitis

Fragrances	Hydroxycitronellal, benzyl salicylate, jasmine absolute, ylang-ylang oil, cananga oil, sandalwood oil, eugenol, cinnamic derivatives, and balsam of Peru
Pigments	D & C Red 31, Red 225; D & C Yellow, No. 11 & 10; and pigments containing phenyl-azo-e-naphthol (PAN), aniline dyes, and kumkum (a red powder commonly used by Hindu women)
Optical whiteners	
Coal tar derivatives	
Bactericidals	Carbanilides like trichlorocarbanilide and Irgasan CF3

and are cosmetic allergens including red and yellow pigments, chromium hydroxide, aniline and azo dyes, bactericidal agents (carbanilides, ricinoleic acids), hair dyes, red kumkum and fragrances [5]. Textile allergens too are common culprits and include optical whiteners, dyes, textile finishes, mercury compounds, formaldehyde, and rubber components. Sometimes occupational allergens like coal tar, pitch, asphalt, mineral oil, and chromates [6].

Clinically, PCD is characterized by reddish-brown to slate grey pigmentation occurring in a reticulate pattern, usually without any active or preceding clinical dermatitis or pruritus thus making the clinical diagnosis difficult in many cases. The skin colour and nature of the allergen can modify the clinical picture. There may be subtle signs of preceding dermatitis in the form of erythema, edema and pruritus in a few patients and some may show positive patch test to cosmetics or their ingredients. The site of dermatitis depends on the allergen responsible; face being the most common site affected in pigmented cosmetic dermatitis [1]. Leow et al. described pigmented contact cheilitis due to ricinoleic acid in lipsticks [7].

Dress or shirt dye dermatitis affects the axillary borders, sparing the vault; and trouser dye dermatitis presents initially on the anterior thigh [1].

Temporal association with cosmetic use and patch test with standard series, cosmetic series, fragrance series and patient's personal product help in finding the causative agent. Photopatch test may be warranted for further evaluation. A majority of the cosmetic allergy cases occurs due to either preservatives (32%) or fragrances (27%). Patch testing with Balsam of Peru and fragrance mix will probably detect over 90% of the cases with fragrance allergy. If a patient is tested positive with a fragrance mix, patch testing with individual agent should be carried out. The concentration of allergen of cosmetic series may too low to induce reaction on back that may result in negative or equivocal patch test, in such cases provocative use test or repeated open application test (ROAT) can be performed. The suspected product is rubbed into the antecubital skin or affected area twice daily for 4–5 days and skin is examined for redness, dryness, and itching. Skin biopsy typically is not required unless there is an unusual presentation. The histology shows damage to the cells of the basal layer hydropic degeneration (localized or complete destruction) and incontinence of pigment [1].

The common differential diagnoses include melasma, lichen planus pigmentosus and exogenous ochronosis. Melasma is very common in constitutionally darker skin types being most common in people with light brown skin. The women of reproductive age group are mostly affected. It is characterized by symmetrical brown to grey brown macules, which may be blotchy, irregular, arcuate, or polycyclic distributed predominantly on the sun exposed areas such as the face (malar, periorbital and perioral area, nose), 'V' area of the neck and forearms. Epidermal melasma presents as brown pigmentation with irregular well defined margins while dermal melasma have greyish pigmentation with poorly defined margins. Some patients may have mixed presentation. Usually there is no history of application of any cosmetic or inflammatory reaction. Lichen planus pigmentosus (LPP) mimics PCD closely and is characterized by asymptomatic diffuse dark-brown to slate-gray macules present mostly over exposed areas and flexures. It affects young individuals with no gender predilection. The face and neck are primarily involved sites but the axilla, inframammary region and groin may also get involved. Exogenous ochronosis (EO), a rare complication of topically applied phenolic intermediates, such as hydroqui-nine (HQ), develops after prolonged use of HQ in high con-centrations in dark-skinned patients. Clinically, it presents as gray-brown or bluish-black macules over the zygomatic regions with less frequent involvement of nasal, peribuccal, and chin areas. Biopsy shows banana-shaped yellow-brown granules in and around collagen bundles along with giant cells and melanophage rich granulomas. Improvement occurs only very slowly (if at all) on withdrawal of HQ [1].

Complete avoidance of the suspected allergen is necessary, and removal of these agents often leads to gradual improve-ment. The patient should also be advised to avoid peak hours of sun exposure. The use of broad rimmed hats and applica-tion of broad spectrum sunscreen over exposed part of body is also recommended. Topical treatments include hydroqui-none, retinoids, and azelaic acid. In addition, chemical peels such as glycolic acid in low concentration and light-based therapy like intense pulsed-light therapy, Q-switched Nd:YAG lasers, and other lasers with wavelengths that specifically tar-get the hyperpigmentation have been found to be useful [8].

Key Points
- Pigmented contact dermatitis is a non-eczematous variant of contact dermatitis which is clinically characterized by hyperpigmentation with little or no signs of dermatitis.
- Pigmented contact dermatitis on the covered area cannot be cured by the application of corticosteroid ointments.
- Pigmented contact dermatitis is caused by various contact allergens from textiles, cosmetic creams, soaps or washing powders for textiles.
- Treatment entails finding out the contact allergens by patch test, and avoiding them for a long time.

References

1. Shenoi SD, Rao R. Pigmented contact dermatitis. Indian J Dermatol Venereol Leprol. 2007;73:285–7.
2. Osmundsen PE. Pigmented contact dermatitis. Br J Dermatol. 1970;83:296–301.
3. Nagao S, Iijima S. Light and electron microscopic study of Riehl's melanosis. Possible mode of its pigmentary incontinence. J Cutan Pathol. 1974;1:165–75.
4. Nakayama H, Matsuo S, Hayakawa K, Takashi K, Shigematsu T, Ota S. Pigmented cosmetic dermatitis. Int J Dermatol. 1984;23:299–305.
5. Forester HR, Schwartz L. Industrial dermatitis and melanosis due to photosensitization. Arch Derm Syphilol. 1939;39:55–68.
6. Nakayama H. Pigmented contact dermatitis and chemical depigmentation. In: Rycroft R, Menne T, Frosch P, Lepoittevin J, editors. Textbook of contact dermatitis. 3rd ed. New York: Springer; 2001. p. 319–33.
7. Leow YH, Tan SH, Ng SK. Pigmented contact cheilitis from ricinoleic acid in lipsticks. Contact Dermatitis. 2003;49(1):48–9.
8. On HR, Hong WJ, Roh MR. Low-pulse energy Q-switched Nd:YAG laser treatment for hair-dye-induced Riehl's melanosis. J Cosmet Laser Ther. 2015;17(3):135–8.

Chapter 10
A Middle Aged Woman with Sudden Onset of Hyperpigmented Patch

Md. Zeeshan

A 38-year-old woman with Fitzpatrick skin type IV presented to the outpatient clinic with asymptomatic, non-progressive brown patchy discoloration of face for past 2 months (Fig. 10.1). She was having melasma for which she underwent chemical peeling at a salon by a beautician. During the chemical peeling, she experienced extreme burning sensation, followed by appearance of dusky-red patches. These dusky-red patches on healing left dark brown to black patches. There is no history of similar lesions elsewhere. Rest of the history was non-contributory.

Cutaneous examination revealed multiple, coalescing, ill-defined brown-dark coloured macules and patches on the face involving whole cheek and zygotemporal area with sparing of peri-orbital area. Based on the case description and the photograph, what is your diagnosis?

1. Post-inflammatory hyperpigmentation
2. Lichen planus pigmentosus
3. Erythema dyschromicum perstans
4. Macular amyloidosis

M. Zeeshan (✉)
Patna Medical College and Hospital, Patna, India

© Springer Nature Switzerland AG 2020
S. Kothiwala et al. (eds.), *Clinical Cases in Disorders of Melanocytes*, Clinical Cases in Dermatology,
https://doi.org/10.1007/978-3-030-22757-9_10

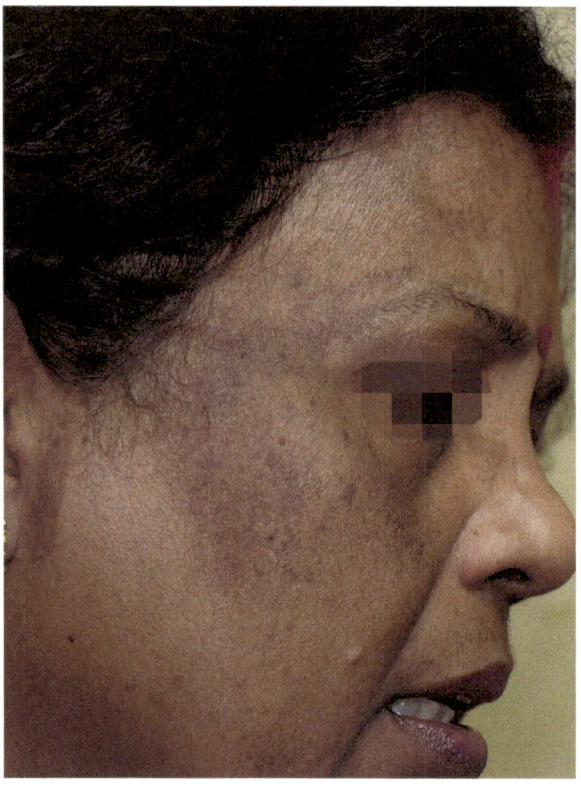

FIGURE 10.1 Dark brown macules and patches on the face in a lady with melasma. Note linear shaped hyperpigmentation in pre-auricular area. (Courtesy: Dr. Piyush Kumar)

Diagnosis

- Postinflammatory hyperpigmentation (PIH)

Discussion

Postinflammatory hyperpigmentation (PIH) is a reactive hypermelanosis that develops following cutaneous inflammation and occurs more commonly in individuals with darker skin (Fitzpatrick skin type IV, and V) [1]. Common causes of PIH include various inflammatory or infectious dermatoses as well as external insults to the skin, such as burn injuries and dermatologic procedures and have been summarized in Table 10.1 [2].

Following certain inflammatory skin diseases, some individuals develop hyperpigmentation, while others develop hypopigmentation, and some individuals may develop both. The severity of PIH is determined by the inherent skin color, degree and depth of inflammation, degree of dermoepidermal junction disruption, and the inflammatory conditions, leading to epidermal and dermal melanin pigment deposition. When there is severe cutaneous inflammation, loss rather than dysfunction of melanocytes occurs, resulting in depigmentation [3].

PIH is clinically characterized by ill-defined brown to blue-gray color macules or patches at the site of a previous inflammatory insult. The brown pigmentation is more of an epidermal melanosis, while in dermal melanosis blue-gray color pigmentation is common [2].

Visual assessment of PIH is generally performed by comparison with the baseline normal skin color. Examination with a Wood's lamp is a simple and useful diagnostic step. Noninvasive objective technologies such as polarized light photography, colorimetry, diffuse reflectance spectroscopy (DRS), hyperspectral imaging (HSI), and reflectance confocal microscopy supplement the clinical assessment and severity and outcome measures of PIH [2]. The histopathology of PIH shows epidermal hypermelanosis and dermal melanophages [1].

The differential diagnosis depends on site and extent of PIH, and common clinical differentials on face include melasma, lichen planus pigmentosus and erythema dyschromicum perstans (shows interface dermatitis on biopsy), and macular amyloidosis. Clinical presentation in melasma is distinct and macular amyloidosis patient shows amyloid deposition in the dermal papillae on biopsy. Erythema dyschromicum perstans is characterized by discrete ash colored macules with

TABLE 10.1 Common dermatologic conditions that can cause postinflammatory hyperpigmentation

---

- **Inflammatory dermatoses**
  Acne/acneiform eruption
  Pseudofolliculitis barbae
  Eczema
  Atopic dermatitis
  Irritant contact dermatitis
  Allergic contact dermatitis
  Pigmented contact dermatitis
  Photoallergic contact dermatitis
  Lichen simplex chronicus
  Insect bites
  Papulosquamous disorders
  Psoriasis
  Pityriasis rosea
  Lichen planus/lichen planus pigmentosus
  Lichenoid dermatitis
  Erythema dyschromicum perstans
  Connective tissue disease
  Lupus erythematosus
  Vasculitis
  Morphea/scleroderma
  Atrophoderma of Pasini and Pierini
  Vesiculobullous disorders
  Pemphigus
  Bullous pemphigoid
  Dermatitis herpetiformis

- **Infections**
  Impetigo
  Viral exanthems
  Chicken pox
  Herpes zoster
  Dermatophytosis
  Syphilis
  Pinta
  Onchocerciasis

- **Cutaneous adverse drug reactions**
  Phototoxic dermatitis
  Morbilliform eruption
  Erythema multiforme
  Fixed drug eruption
  Stevens-Johnson syndrome/Toxic epidermal necrolysis
  Lichenoid drug eruption

- **Dermatological procedures**
  Chemical peel
  Dermabrasion
  Cryotherapy
  Laser treatment
  Intense pulsed light treatment

- **Miscellaneous**
  Mycosis fungoides
  Neurotic excoriation
  Sunburn
  Trauma
  Friction

---

slightly elevated erythematous margins. Lesions gradually coalesce and lose erythematous border to become gray-blue. Common sites are face, neck, arm and trunk. On histopathology, interface dermatitis; vacuolar degeneration of the basal cell layer, pigment incontinence, and perivascular mononuclear cell infiltrate are seen. Lichen planus pigmentosus (LPP) is characterized by slaty-gray to brownish-black pigmentation symmetrically over photo-exposed areas, most commonly face and neck, followed by upper limbs. It have insidious onset and there is no history of preceding inflammation. There is no fixed pattern of pigmentation like post inflammatory hyperpigmentation. The early lesions of LPP show marked inflammation at dermoepidermal junction which later subside, leaving behind dermal pigmentation in older lesion. Macular amyloidosis is a type of primary localized cutaneous amyloidosis which present as dusky brown colored pigmentation in rippled pattern over upper back, arm, forearm and shins. Usually it is associated with itching. Histopathology shows significant pigment incontinence with eosinophilic amorphous depost in papillary dermis [1, 2].

Mainstay of treatment is to address the cause of the inflammation and to practice strict sun protection. Several therapeutic modalities are available for the treatment of PIH, including topical agents, chemical peels, and lasers. Among topical therapies hydroquinone, retinoids [4], azelaic acid, and kojic acid are shown to have role in treatment [5]. Kligman and Willis first used combination therapy as HQ 5%, tretinoin 0.1% and dexamethasone 0.1% in 1975 [6]. Superficial to medium-depth peeling agents such as glycolic acid [7], salicylic acid and Jessner solution are commonly used in the treatment [1]. Among lasers, 1064-nm quality-switched (QS) neodymium-doped yttrium aluminum garnet (Nd:YAG), QS Ruby, and 1550 nm Erbium fiber fractional thermolysis are commonly used in treatment of PIH [5, 8, 9].

Key Points

- Postinflammatory hyperpigmentation (PIH) commonly occurs after various endogenous and exogenous stimuli, especially in dark-skinned individuals.
- The site and extent of pigmentation corresponds to prior inflammation/injury and helps in making a clinical diagnosis. The condition is usually non-progressive.
- Severe inflammation may lead to postinflammatory hypopigmentation or depigmentation. Same patient may develop both postinflammatory hyperpigmentation and hypopigmentation.
- Identifying and avoiding the inflammatory stimulus, and sun protection are the key steps in the management of PIH.

References

1. Taylor S, Grimes P, Lim J, Im S, Lui H. Postinflammatory hyperpigmentation. J Cutan Med Surg. 2009;13:183–91.
2. Silpa-Archa N, Kohli I, Chaowattanapanit S, Lim HW, Hamzavi I. Postinflammatory hyperpigmentation: a comprehensive overview: epidemiology, pathogenesis, clinical presentation, and noninvasive assessment technique. J Am Acad Dermatol. 2017;77(4):591–605.
3. Papa CM, Kligman AM. The behavior of melanocytes in inflammation. J Invest Dermatol. 1965;45:465–73.
4. Ortonne JP. Retinoid therapy of pigmentary disorders. Dermatol Ther. 2006;19:280–8.
5. Chaowattanapanit S, Silpa-Archa N, Kohli I, Lim HW, Hamzavi I. Postinflammatory hyperpigmentation: a comprehensive overview: treatment options and prevention. J Am Acad Dermatol. 2017;77(4):607–21.
6. Kligman AM, Willis I. A new formula for depigmenting human skin. Arch Dermatol. 1975;111:40–8.
7. Grover C, Reddu BS. The therapeutic value of glycolic acid peels in dermatology. Indian J Dermatol Venereol Leprol. 2003;69:148–50.

8. Tafazzoli A, Rostan EF, Goldman MP. Q-switched ruby laser treatment for postsclerotherapy hyperpigmentation. Dermatol Surg. 2000;26:653–6.
9. Tse Y, Levine VJ, McClain SA, Ashinoff R. The removal of cutaneous pigmented lesions with the Q-switched ruby laser and the Q-switched neodymium: yttrium-aluminum-garnet laser. A comparative study. J Dermatol Surg Oncol. 1994;20:795–800.

Chapter 11
Itchy Pigmented Lesions on the Upper Back

Niharika Ranjan Lal

A 40-year-old lady presented with the complaints of itching and hyperpigmentation of upper back and upper extremities of 2 years duration. Patient started to develop mild itching over upper back and lateral aspect of arms; then gradually she noticed hyperpigmentation on sites of itching. Since last one year she noticed similar lesions over bilateral shins. She gave history of chronic use of loofah for rubbing soap during bath. Rest of the history was non-contributory and there was no history of any dermatoses or drug intake prior to onset of lesions. On examination, she had patchy dusky brown-grey small macules, coalescing to form bigger patches, upper back (Fig. 11.1) and arms symmetrically (Fig. 11.2). At some places, macules were showing "rippled pattern" of arrangement (vide Fig. 11.2). Based on the history and examination, what is your diagnosis?

1. Lichen planus pigmentosus
2. Notalgia paresthetica
3. Macular amyloidosis
4. Poikiloderma of civatte

N. R. Lal (✉)
ESI PGIMSR and ESI Medical College, Kolkata, India

© Springer Nature Switzerland AG 2020
S. Kothiwala et al. (eds.), *Clinical Cases in Disorders of Melanocytes*, Clinical Cases in Dermatology,
https://doi.org/10.1007/978-3-030-22757-9_11

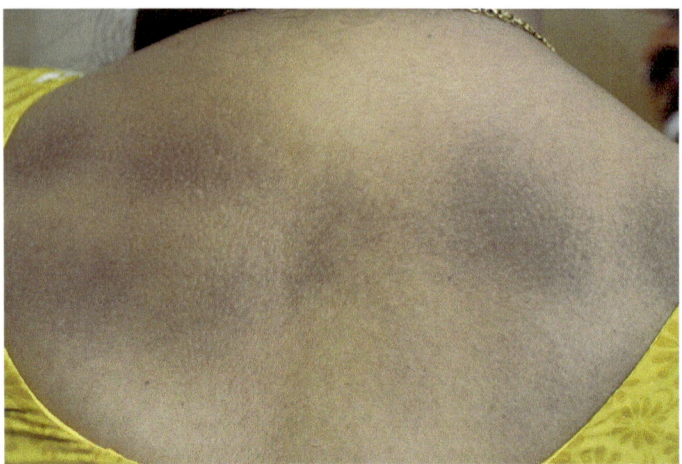

FIGURE 11.1 Multiple hyperpigmented patches on upper back

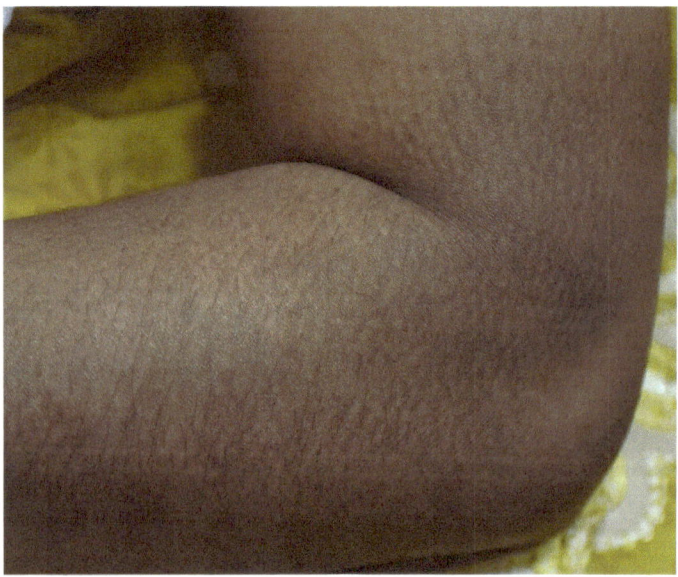

FIGURE 11.2 Multiple hyperpigmented macules arranged in a "rippled pattern"

Diagnosis

• Macular amyloidosis

Itchy, hyperpigmented macules in a rippled pattern on the upper back is clinically diagnostic of macular amyloidosis. Dermoscopy is non-invasive diagnostic tool and can be used to diagnose macular amyloidosis with certainty. Dermoscopy shows the presence of brown clods with radiating brown lines, in a "Hub and Spoke" pattern (Fig. 11.3).

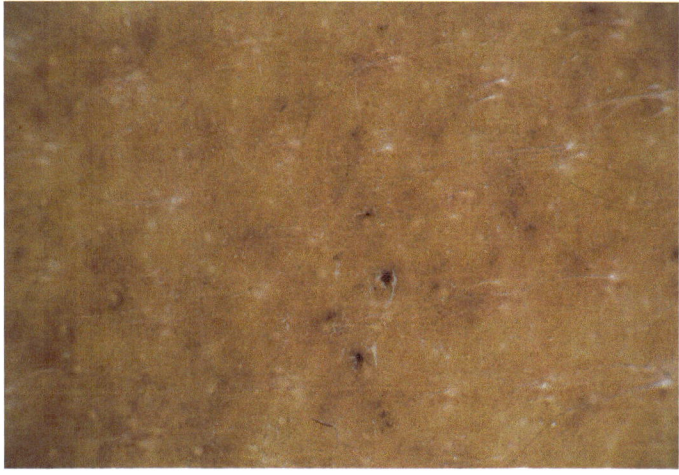

FIGURE 11.3 Dermoscopy of the back lesion showing brown clods with radiating brown lines, in a "Hub and Spoke" pattern (Courtesy: Dr. Shekhar Neema)

Discussion

The term "amyloid", which stands for starch-like (Latin *amylum*) was introduced in science by Rudolph Virchow in 1854. The key feature of all types of amyloidosis is extracellular deposition of autologous proteins as characteristic amyloid fibril [1].

Macular amyloidosis (MA) represents a common variant of primary localized cutaneous amyloidosis (PLCA). The deposition of amyloid in previously apparently normal skin without deposits in the internal organs is known as primary localised cutaneous amyloidosis (PLCA). It is rare in western population, but has a high incidence in South-east Asia and some South American populations. Various subtypes of PLCA are recognized, including the more common macular and papular (lichen amyloidosis) types and the rare forms like the nodular variety and amylodosis dyschromia cutis. Both macular and papular lesions may occur in the same patient giving rise to biphasic amyloidosis [2]. Among all PLCA, only nodular amyloidosis has been found to be associated with systemic amyloidosis in 15–50% of patients and hence, long term follow-up of patients with nodular amyloidosis is recommended [3].

Multiple factors may play a collective role in the genesis of macular amyloidosis. These include racial, familial, and environmental factors, atopy, sunlight, friction, and female gender [4]. Amyloid deposits have also been shown to contain disulfide bonds, which are present in keratin. Based on this finding and on those of ultra-structural studies, cutaneous amyloid deposits are thought to be derived from degenerated keratin peptides of apoptotic keratinocytes transformed into amyloid fibrils by dermal macrophages and fibroblasts. A working hypothesis is that the epidermal trauma induced by long term scratching and rubbing results in keratinocyte degradation and formation of amyloid. Additionally, immunofluorescence studies with antikeratin antiserum have shown intense staining of the amyloid for the antikeratin antibody [5].

Clinically, MA presents as poorly delineated hyperpigmented patches consisting of grayish-brown macules, sometimes arranged in a "rippled pattern." The most commonly involved sites are the interscapular area, and extensors of extremities (arms, shins and forearms), although involvement of the clavicles, breast, face, auricular concha, neck, and axilla have also been reported. It is usually pruritic (82%) and the degree of itching varies from mild to severe. It follows a chronic, progressive course with increasing pigmentation and extent of involvement. Other common PLCA is lichen amyloidosis which presents with intensely pruritic, discrete or coalescing, hyperkeratotic papules noted most commonly on the anterior tibiae. However, extensive lesions may involve extensor surfaces of the upper extremities and trunk. Amyloidosis cutis dyschromica is a rare type of PLCA characterized by the presence of both hyper- and hypopigmentation or depigmentation in reticular pattern distributed all over body [1].

Diagnosis of MA is made by its clinical presentation, dermoscopy, and histopathology. Histopathology with hematoxylin and eosin stain shows significant pigment incontinence with eosinophilic, amorphous deposits in papillary dermis which stain positive for amyloid with Congo red stain. Under polarized light, it gives green birefringence [5].

The common clinical differentials include lichen planus pigmentosus (LPP), notalgia paresthetica (NP) and poikiloderma of Civatte. LPP is clinically characterised by symmetrical distribution of dark brown to gray or gray-blue, round or oval macules with irregular and poorly-defined borders, which eventually enlarge and coalesce. It may be associated with variable itching and affects both sun-exposed and sun-protected areas of the body. Absence of rippled pattern helps in ruling out it as differential of macular amyloidosis. Histology reveals features similar to lichen planus with basal cell vacuolization and band like infiltrate at dermo-epidermal junction [6]. NP is a sensory neuropathy caused by entrapment of the posterior rami of spinal nerves T2 through T6 affecting the interscapular area and is associated with pain, paresthesia, hyperesthesia, or hypoesthesia rather than pruritus [7]. Poikiloderma of Civatte affects sun exposed areas in light skinned, perimenopausal females manifested by pink to brownish reticular patches consisting of linear telangiectasia, mottled hyperpigmentation and superficial atrophy. It affects the sides of neck, peripheral face and upper chest. Histology shows thinning of epidermis and solar elastosis in papillary dermis [8].

Treatment of MA is often disappointing. Topical treatment with corticosteroids with or without occlusion, 10% dimethylsulphoxide (DMSO), retinoids have been tried, but results are often unsatisfactory. Etretinate and acitretin therapy has been beneficial in some cases, but the condition seems to relapse after the treatment is stopped [9]. Dermabrasion may be beneficial on lichen amyloidosis of the shins. Oral cyclophosphamide and cyclosporine have a limited therapeutic efficacy [10]. In a study by Ostovari et al., 90% of patients with MA demonstrated more than 50% reduction in their pigmentation with the Q-switched Nd-YAG laser [11]. Ten and twenty percent trichloroacetic acid peels have also been tried with more than 50% improvement [9].

Key Points

- Macular amyloidosis is a type of primary localised cutaneous amyloidosis in which amyloid deposit occurs in skin without involving internal organs.
- Genetic and environmental factors result in focal epidermal damage with subsequent conversion of degenerated epidermal cell into amyloid in the papillary dermis which stain positive with Congo red.
- Multiple small dusky brown-grey hyperpigmented macules arranged in rippled pattern is characteristic of macular amyloidosis.
- Various treatment modalities have been tried with modest success.

References

1. Bandhlish A, Aggarwal A, Koranne RV. A clinico-epidemiological study of macular amyloidosis from north India. Indian J Dermatol. 2012;57(4):269–74.
2. Mehrotra K, Dewan R, Kumar JV, Dewan A. Primary cutaneous amyloidosis: a clinical, histopathological and immunofluorescence study. J Clin Diagn Res. 2017;11(8):WC01–5.
3. Steciuk A, Dompmartin A, Troussard X, Verneuil L, Macro M, Comoz F, et al. Cutaneous amyloidosis and possible association with systemic amyloidosis. Int J Dermatol. 2002;41(3):127–32.
4. Eswaramoorthy V, Kaur I, Das A, Kumar B. Macular amyloidosis: etiological factors. J Dermatol. 1999;26:305–10.
5. Vijaya B, Dalal BS, Sunila, Manjunath GV. Primary cutaneous amyloidosis: a clinico-pathological study with emphasis on polarized microscopy. Indian J Pathol Microbiol. 2012;55:170–4.
6. Robles-Méndez JC, Rizo-Frías P, Herz-Ruelas ME, Pandya AG, Ocampo Candiani J. Lichen planus pigmentosus and its variants: review and update. Int J Dermatol. 2018;57:505–14.
7. Howard M, Sahhar L, Andrews F, Bergman R, Gin D. Notalgia paresthetica: a review for dermatologists. Int J Dermatol. 2018;57(4):388–92.
8. Katoulis AC, Stavrianeas NG, Panayiotides JG, Bozi E, Vamvasakis E, Kalogeromitros D, et al. Poikiloderma of Civatte: a histopathological and ultrastructural study. Dermatology. 2007;214(2):177–82.
9. Weidner T, Illing T, Elsner P. Primary localized cutaneous amyloidosis: a systematic treatment review. Am J Clin Dermatol. 2017;18(5):629–42.
10. Das J, Gogoi RK. Treatment of primary localised cutaneous amyloidosis with cyclophosphamide. Indian J Dermatol Venereol Leprol. 2003;69:163–4.
11. Ostovari N, Mohtasham N, Oadras MS, Malekzad F. 532-nm and 1064-nm Q-switched Nd:YAG laser therapy for reduction of pigmentation in macular amyloidosis patches. J Eur Acad Dermatol Venereol. 2008;22:442–6.

Chapter 12
A Young Man with Mottled Pigmentation on Trunk

Piyush Kumar

A 27-year-old male, from rural area of West Bengal, presented with progressive, asymptomatic, pigmentation of the trunk of 5 years duration, and rough palm and soles of 2 years duration. He developed both hyperpigmented and hypopigmented flat lesions on upper back 5 years back which had progressed to involve the trunk completely. He started developing small, rough, solid elevated lesions on the palms and soles 2 years back. These lesions had been increasing in number since then and were coalescing to form bigger lesions. The lesions were asymptomatic, but interfere with walking and manual activities with hand. Also, he complained of slight breathlessness on exertion. Two of his family members and many persons from his neighborhood were suffering from similar skin lesions, though of different degree of involvement. On enquiring, people in his locality were drinking groundwater without processing. On dermatological examination, there was diffuse hyperpigmentation of the trunk, along with multiple hyperpigmented as well as hypopigmented macules. Additionally, a few hyperpigmented, hyperkeratotic papules and plaques were noted (Fig. 12.1). Palm and soles were notable for the presence of discrete as well as

P. Kumar (✉)
Katihar Medical College and Hospital, Katihar, India

© Springer Nature Switzerland AG 2020
S. Kothiwala et al. (eds.), *Clinical Cases in Disorders of Melanocytes*, Clinical Cases in Dermatology,
https://doi.org/10.1007/978-3-030-22757-9_12

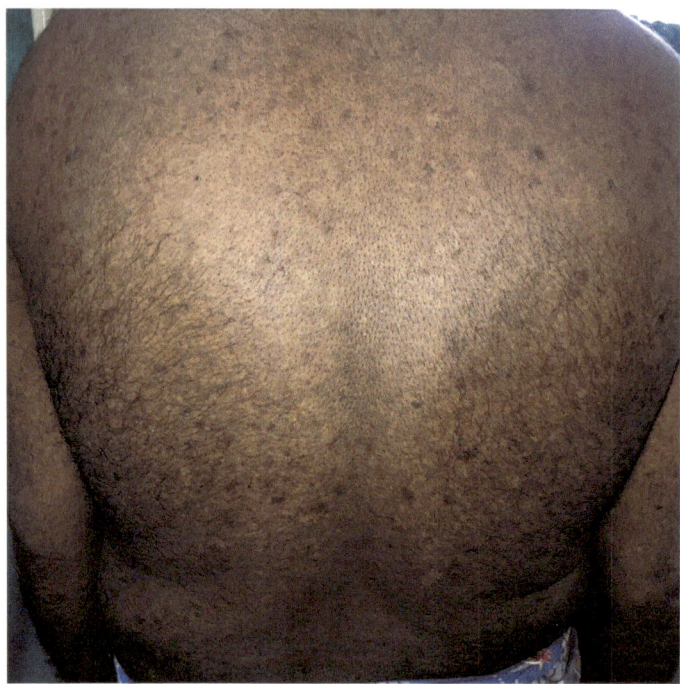

FIGURE 12.1 Multiple hyperpigmented as well as hypopigmented macules on the back. There are a few lesions of arsenical keratoses too. (Courtesy: Dr. Anirban Das)

confluent hyperkeratotic papules (Fig. 12.2). Rest of the mucocutaneous examination was non-contributory. Patient was referred to pulmonologist and internist for the evaluation of breathlessness. Based on clinical presentation, what is your diagnosis?

1. Pigmented xerodermoid
2. Pityriasis versicolor
3. Dowling Degos disease
4. Chronic arsenicosis

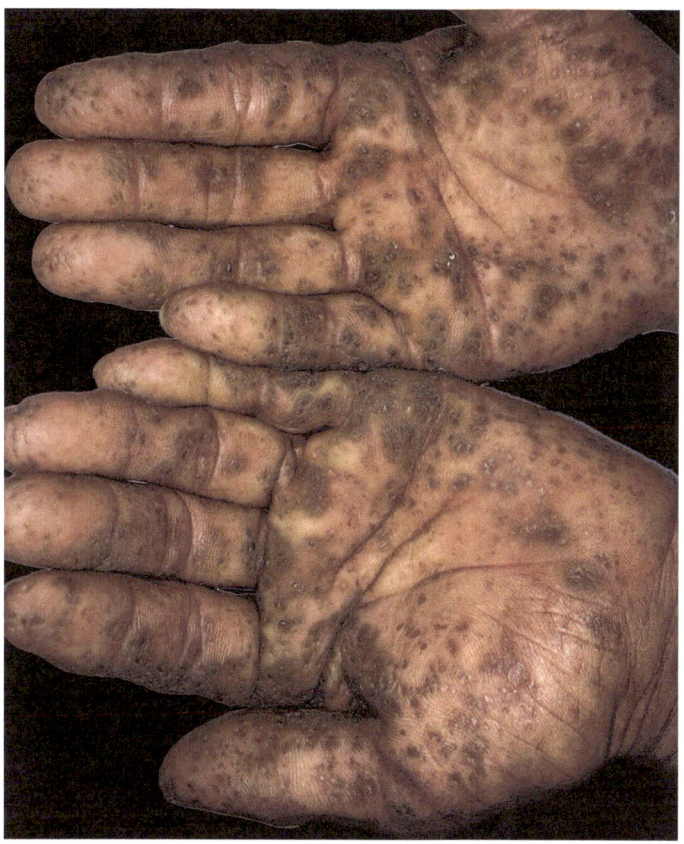

FIGURE 12.2 Multiple discrete and confluent keratotic papules present bilaterally on palms (Courtesy: Dr. Anirban Das)

Diagnosis

- Chronic arsenicosis

The clinical presentation (both hyperpigmented and hypopigmented macules and patches of covered parts along with hyperkeratotic lesions on palms and soles) was characteristic of chronic arsenicosis. Further confirmation was done by demonstrating higher level of arsenic in urine (84 µg/L), and drinking water (132 ppb).

Discussion

Arsenicosis is a chronic multisystem disorder resulting from high level of arsenic in the body. Though cases have been reported from many parts of the world, the two worst affected areas in the world are Bangladesh and West Bengal, India. Arsenic exposure may occur from inhalation, and absorption through the skin, but is mostly by ingestion of contaminated drinking water. Other sources of arsenic include agricultural pesticides and herbicides; fungicides and insecticides; wood preservatives; paints; cosmetics; and manufacture of semiconductors, light emitting diodes, lasers and microwave circuits [1]. Chronic arsenicosis may be seen in sheep dip workers, in vineyard workers using arsenical pesticides, and from drinking contaminated wine. Additionally, arsenic is present as a contaminant in many traditional remedies and long term ingestion of such medicines may cause the disease [2].

After ingestion, arsenic is mainly absorbed in small intestine and is metabolized in liver and excreted in urine. Arsenic is consumed mainly in two forms, arsenite (As +3) and arsenate (As +5). Arsenite (As 3+) binds with sulfhydryl groups in keratin filament and has a tendency to accumulate in the skin, hair, nails, and mucosae of the oral cavity, esophagus, stomach, and the small intestine. On the other hand, arsenate (As +5) is predominantly deposited in the skeleton. Arsenic, mostly the arsenite (As +3) form, binds with the sulfhydryl groups present in various essential compounds, e.g., glutathione (GSH), cysteine, and exerts its toxicity by inactivating up to 200 enzymes, especially those involved in cellular energy pathways, and DNA synthesis and repair. Arsenate (As +5) in addition to getting converted into arsenite (As +3) form, causes toxicity by 'arsenolysis'in which it replaces phosphate during glycolysis, resulting in ineffective generation of adenosine triphosphate (ATP). Other mechanisms include generation of reactive oxygen intermediates and metabolic activation processes causing lipid peroxidation and DNA damage. Arsenic induced carcinogenesis is believed to result from hypermethylation of DNA, particularly of the promoter region, resulting in inactivation of the tumor suppressor genes [3].

No system is spared in chronic arsenicosis, but skin is the most predominantly affected organ. The cutaneous manifestations are of diagnostic value and include pigmentary changes; keratotic papules and plaques; and various cutaneous malignancies. The pigmentary changes are reported to be the earliest and the commonest of all dermatological manifestations. The pigmentation can be diffuse (with trunk being affected most severely) or localized affecting skin folds. Another common pattern of pigmentation is fine hyperpigmented macules, known as 'rain-drop pigmentation'. Simultaneously, depigmented macules appear on normal skin or hyperpigmented background resulting in a distinctive appearance of 'leucomelanosis'. Pigmentary changes is noted in mucosa too and blotchy pigmentation affecting the undersurface of the tongue or buccal mucosa is common. Another important examination finding is Mee's lines (transverse bands of true leukonychia) in the fingernails and toenails [3].

Arsenical hyperkeratosis characteristically affects the palms and soles, and the involvement is graded as mild, moderate, or severe depending on the extent and severity. In the early stages of keratosis (i.e., the mild variety), the involved skin has an indurated, gritty feel with papules less than 2 mm in size. In the moderate variety, the lesions advance to form punctate, wartlike keratoses >2–5 mm in size. When the keratosis becomes severe, it may form keratotic elevations more than 5 mm in size and become confluent and diffuse. Keratotic papules may noted on dorsa of the extremities and trunk too [4].

The development of various cutaneous malignancies in chronic arsenicosis is quite common and may occur in the hyperkeratotic areas, as well normal appearing skin of the trunk, extremities, or head. The affected patients have a tendency to develop multiple lesions simultaneously or over a long period of time and lesions usually appear on the covered parts. Arsenic exposure has been associated with three types of skin cancers mainly—Bowen's disease, basal cell carcinoma and squamous cell carcinoma [3].

The prominent systemic manifestations have been summarized in Table 12.1 [4].

The common differential diagnoses for leukomelanosis include pityriasis versicolor, Xeroderma pigmentosum and pigmented xerodermoid, and Dowling Degos disease and have been summarized in Table 12.2. The clinical differentials for diffuse pigmentation include Addison's disease and vitamin B12 deficiency among others. Occurrence of multiple cutaneous and systemic malignancies warrants consideration of various cancer predisposition syndromes.

Cutaneous manifestations (melanosis, keratosis, and cutaneous cancers) are specific enough to allow a trained dermatologists or arsenic experts to clinically confirm a case even without laboratory backup. The laboratory confirmation of diagnosis rests on demonstrating elevated level of arsenic in drinking water consumed by patient and in urine, hair and nail samples from patient. The maximum permissible limit of arsenic in drinking water as per the recent guideline of World Health Organization (WHO) is 10 ppb. However, many developing countries have chosen 50 ppb as cut-off limit. The arsenic concentration of 1 mg/kg in hair and 1.5 mg/kg in nails have been shown to correlate with clinical disease in chronic arsenicosis. Urine arsenic >50 μg/L indicated continued exposure [4, 5].

There is no specific treatment for chronic arsenicosis and hence, the principal focus of management is on prevention of the problem. Raising public awareness by information, education, and communication strategies are important tools for prevention. Once the diagnosis is made, absolute cessation of exposure to contaminated drinking water is needed. The patient is then offered various supportive measures and periodic follow up to early detect cancers. Hyperkeratotic lesions are treated by keratolytics (5–10% salicylic acid and 10–20% urea) and retinoids. Early diagnosis and excision of skin cancers is advocated. Symptomatic treatment is offered to patients with cardiovascular, gastrointestinal, respiratory and nervous system manifestations. Periodic life-long surveillance for detection of cancer in chronic arsenicosis patients is an

TABLE 12.1 Systemic manifestations in chronic arsenicosis

System	Pathomechanism	Manifestations
Cardiovascular system	Generalized atherosclerosis Myocardial injury, cardiac arrhythmias, and cardiomyopathy	Ischemic heart disease, blackfoot disease, hypertension, cerebrovascular disease, and carotid atherosclerosis
Gastrointestinal system	Hepatic fibrosis	Gastric symptoms, including nausea, loss of appetite, constipation, or sometimes diarrhea, noncirrhotic portal fibrosis, hepatomegaly
Central nervous system		Changes in behaviour, confusion, and memory loss. Cognitive impairment
Peripheral nervous system	Distal axonopathy with axonal degeneration, especially of large myelinated fibers of both sensory and motor neurons	Peripheral neuropathy (sensory features were more common than motor features), essentially paresthesias (viz., burning, tingling sensations), pain, and tenderness in the affected limb with or without distal limb weakness and atrophy; and absent or diminished tendon reflexes
Respiratory system	Oxidative stress	Cough, shortness of breath with the breath sounds revealing crepitations and/ or rhonchi
Urogenital system	Renal tubular necrosis, nephritis and nephrosis	Urine may be red or green in color, dysuria and anuria Renal tubular necrosis
Hematological system		Anemia, leucopenia, and thrombocytopenia
Pregnant mothers	Vasculopathy	Spontaneous abortions, stillbirths, preterm births; and high perinatal and neonatal mortality
Carcinogenicity	DNA damage	Skin, lung, bladder, kidney, prostate, liver, uterus, and possibly lymphatic tissues

TABLE 12.2 Differential diagnosis of leukomelanosis of chronic arsenicosis [4]

Disease	Key features
Pityriasis versicolor	The perifollicular macules coalesce to form bigger lesions. The lesions may be mildly scaly and may be itchy. KOH mount of the skin scrapings confirm the diagnosis
Xeroderma pigmentosum	The affected patients develop pigmentary changes since infancy and cutaneous malignancies on exposed parts since early childhood. Also, patients complaints of photosensitivity and develop corneal ulcers and subsequent opacity
Pigmented xerodermoid	A milder form of xeroderma pigmentosum in which affected patients do not develop serious manifestations like corneal ulcers and cutaneous malignancies
Dowling Degos disease	Dowling-Degos disease is an autosomal dominant genodermatosis, characterised by reticulate pigmentation of the flexures, comedo-like papules and perioral pitted scars

absolute necessity. Treatment with chelating agents like dimercaptosuccinic acid (DMSA), dimercaptopropane succinate (DMPS), and d-penicillamine has been considered; however, their utility in routine management of chronic arsenicosis is yet to be established [6].

Key Points
- Chronic arsenicosis acquired by drinking contaminated drinking water has been recognized in many countries, but is most common in Bangladesh and India.
- Chronic arsenicosis can be diagnosed clinically by characteristic skin findings- pigmentation of the trunk and keratotic papules on the palms and soles.
- There is increased risk of developing various malignancies, including cutaneous malignancies of the covered parts.

Hence, lifelong surveillance is required to diagnose cancers at an early stage.

- There is no definitive treatment for chronic arsenicosis and manifestations may progress even after cessation of further exposure to arsenic. Prevention is the best tool available to fight this disease.

References

1. Ghosh P, Roy C, Das NK, Sengupta SR. Epidemiology and prevention of chronic arsenicosis: an Indian perspective. Indian J Dermatol Venereol Leprol. 2008;74:582–93.
2. Khandpur S, Malhotra AK, Bhatia V, Gupta S, Sharma VK, Mishra R, Arora NK. Chronic arsenic toxicity from ayurvedic medicines. Int J Dermatol. 2008;47(6):618–21.
3. Sengupta SR, Das NK, Datta PK. Pathogenesis, clinical features and pathology of chronic arsenicosis. Indian J Dermatol Venereol Leprol. 2008;74:559–70.
4. Das A, Paul R, Das NK. Chronic arsenicosis: clinical features and diagnosis. In: Chakrabarty N, editor. Arsenic toxicity: prevention and treatment. 1st ed. Boca Raton: CRC Press; 2015. p. 376–400.
5. Das NK, Sengupta SR. Arsenicosis: diagnosis and treatment. Indian J Dermatol Venereol Leprol. 2008;74:571–81.
6. Kumar P, Paul R, Sil A, Das NK. Management of chronic arsenicosis: an overview. In: Chakrabarty N, editor. Arsenic toxicity: prevention and treatment. 1st ed. Boca Raton: CRC Press; 2015. p. 401–28.

Chapter 13
A Young Man with Generalized Pigmentation

Divya Sachdev, Piyush Kumar, and Panchami Debbarman

A 30-years-old unmarried male presented with complaints of generalized weakness, loosening of clothes and progressive pigmentation for the last 6 months. He had no history of tightening of skin, loose stools/steatorrhea, seizure disorder, tuberculosis or any drug intake prior to onset of pigmentation. There was no history of similar illness in the family. He is non-alcoholic, non-smoker and follows a vegetarian diet. On general examination, he was of thin and malnourished built, and had dry and lustreless hair with angular cheilitis, atrophic glossitis, and pallor. Cutaneous examination revealed generalized hyperpigmentation especially of the sun-exposed areas, flexural folds, and skin creases, including the creases on the palms (Figs. 13.1 and 13.2). Oral mucosa too showed isolated hyperpigmented patches (Fig. 13.3) Serum electrolyte and thyroid profile tests were within normal limits. Blood picture revealed macrocytic anemia with hemoglobin 9.8 g/dL, mean corpuscular volume 114 fL, erythrocyte

D. Sachdev (✉)
Consultant Dermatologist, Raipur, India

P. Kumar
Katihar Medical College and Hospital, Katihar, India

P. Debbarman
Consultant Dermatologist, Mumbai, India

© Springer Nature Switzerland AG 2020
S. Kothiwala et al. (eds.), *Clinical Cases in Disorders of Melanocytes*, Clinical Cases in Dermatology,
https://doi.org/10.1007/978-3-030-22757-9_13

103

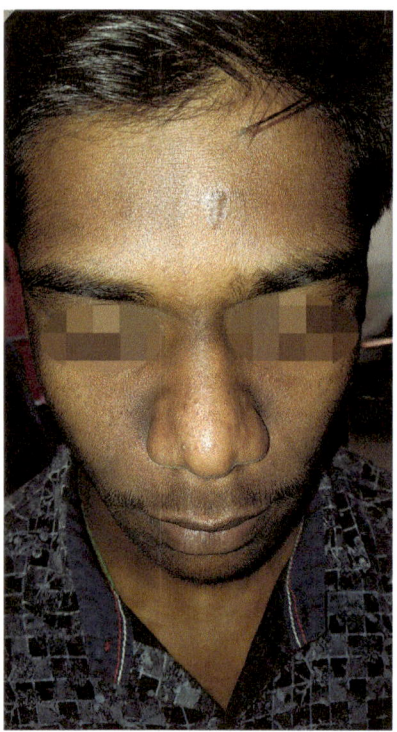

FIGURE 13.1 Pigmentation of the face in vitamin B12 deficiency

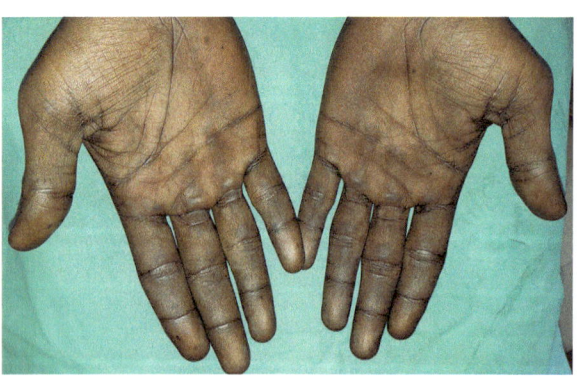

FIGURE 13.2 Pigmentation of the palms in vitamin B12 deficiency. Note pigmentation of palmar creases

sedimentation rate 55 mm at the end of first hour and total leukocyte count 5900/μL. Bone marrow examination did not reveal any abnormality. Serum morning cortisol done in response to insulin stress test was 16.77 μg/dL (normal range − 7–28 μg/dL).

Based on the case description and photographs, what is your diagnosis?

1. Addison's disease
2. Vitamin B12 deficiency
3. Cushing's Disease
4. Laugier-Hunziker Syndrome

Diagnosis

• Vitamin B12 deficiency

Discussion

Diffuse hyperpigmentation may have a systemic cause of which vitamin B12 deficiency is one of the rare causes. The body reserve of vitamin B12 ranges from 2000 to 3000 μg which doesn't need replenishment for the next 3–4 years and hence, vitamin B12 deficiency does not manifest until and unless deficiency persists for a long time [1]. Common cause of vitamin B 12 deficiency is malabsorption, usually due to pernicious anemia or gastric resection and rarely, due to inadequate intake [2]. Inadequate intake almost exclusively occurs in strict vegetarians as vitamin B12 is naturally found in animal products like meat, eggs, fish, poultry, milk and milk products [3].

Vitamin B12 is needed as a cofactor for enzymes like methionine synthase (cytoplasmic) and methylmalonyl coenzyme A mutase (mitochondrial). Also, Cobalamin is essential for DNA synthesis, haematopoiesis and myelination. As a result, vitamin B12 deficiency presents with different combinations of neurological manifestations (peripheral neuropathy, subacute combined degeneration of the spinal cord,

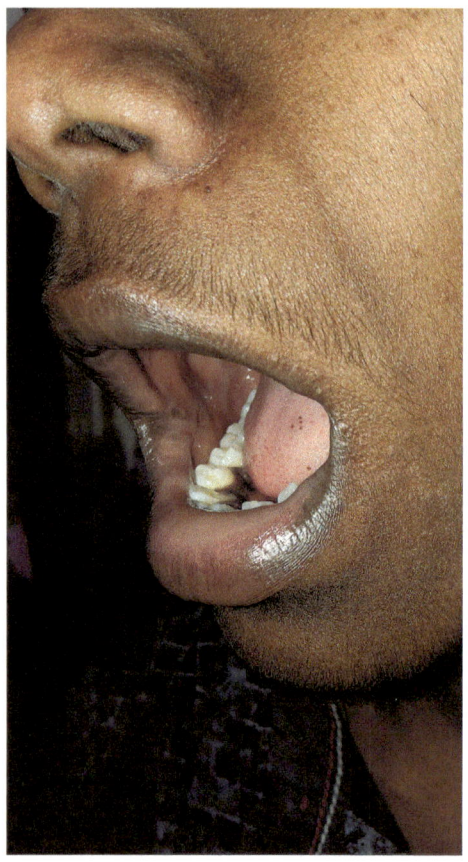

FIGURE 13.3 Mucosal pigmentation in vitamin B12 deficiency

ataxia), hematological changes (megaloblastic anemia and pancytopenia), psychiatric (psychosis, depression, mania and dementia), gastrointestinal (diarrhea), dermatologic (discoloration of skin, hair and nails), cardiovascular manifestations (thrombosis, myocardial infarction, stroke and syncope), and optic atrophy [4]. Neurological manifestations are common presenting features and the commonest neurological signs are diminished vibration sense and proprioception in the legs and can include impaired distal cutaneous sensation. Limb reflexes may be exaggerated, diminished, or absent depending on the relative involvement of the cord. Lateral column signs of a spastic paraparesis may occur, accompanied by autonomic bladder, bowel, or sexual symptoms [5].

Cutaneous manifestations associated with vitamin B12 deficiency are characteristic and include skin hyperpigmentation, angular stomatitis, and hair changes like premature canitis. Most common type of cutaneous manifestation is reversible brown to black pigmentation over the dorsum of hands and feet (predominantly over knuckles and interphalangeal joints; and palmar creases) and over pressure points like elbows, knees and malleoli. Other sites of pigmentation include sun exposed areas, genital, perineum, and umbilicus, resembling addisonian type of pigmentation. Rarely, hyperpigmentation of skin may be the only presenting manifestation of vitamin B12 deficiency and awareness of this condition may lead to early diagnosis [6]. Hyperpigmentation in vitamin B12 deficiency is related to depletion of glutathione which increases the activity of tyrosinase and increases eumelanogenesis, resulting clinically in hyperpigmentation. Ultraviolet rays cause further depletion of intracellular glutathione, thereby accentuating the pigmentation in sun-exposed areas. Mucosal manifestation may vary from mucosal pigmentation, mucositis, glossodynia to recurrent ulcerations. The classic manifestation of mucous involvement is Hunter glossitis/Moeller glossitis (25% cases) that has an early inflammatory stage presenting as red beefy tongue and a late atrophic stage causing atrophy of papillae [5].

It is important to note that folate deficiency may present with similar melanosis of skin and neurological manifestations. Sometimes, folate and vitamin B12 deficiencies may co-exist in same patient and it is prudent to supplement both when deficiency of either nutrient is suspected. Both Folate and vitamin B12 have essential roles in methionine synthase mediated conversion of homocysteine to methionine, which is essential for nucleotide synthesis and genomic and non-genomic methylation Folate deficiency manifests as fatigue, weakness, headaches, difficulty concentrating, palpitations and diarrhoea similar to vitamin B12 deficiency. In the early stages, the tongue may be red and painful leading to a smooth shiny surface in the chronic stages of deficiency. The reported neuropsychiatric effects of folate deficiency are remarkably similar to those described for vitamin B12 deficiency [7].

The common differential diagnoses include Addison's disease, Cushing's disease and Laugier-Hunziker syndrome. Addison's disease results from adrenal insufficiency caused by a defect anywhere in the hypothalamic-pituitary-adrenal axis. Patients present with generalized hyperpigmentation and the diagnosis is confirmed by estimating serum electrolytes and serum 8 a.m. cortisol level. Cushing's disease is caused by prolonged exposure to elevated levels of glucocorticoids (endogenous or exogenous). Patients develop proximal muscle weakness, easy bruising, weight gain, hirsutism, and, in children, growth retardation, hypertension, osteopenia, diabetes mellitus, and impaired immune function. Addisonian pattern of pigmentation is noted in 10% patients. Besides cutaneous and systemic changes nails shows longitudinal pigmented bands and hair is often dark. The diagnosis of requires demonstration of inappropriately high level of cortisol in the serum or urine and screening tests include midnight serum or salivary cortisol, 24-h urine free cortisol and low dose dexamethasone suppression test. Laugier-Hunziker syndrome is an acquired pigmentary disorder presenting with hyperpigmented macules of the lips and buccal mucosa with associated longitudinal melanonychia, without any systemic features [5].

A diagnosis of vitamin B12 deficiency is often overlooked in its early stages because these signs are not specific to vitamin B12 deficiency alone. Vitamin B12 deficiency results in megaloblastic anemia and pancytopenia- so patients have low hemoglobin, low total leucocyte count and reticulocyte count, but high mean corpuscular volume. Vitamin B12 level estimation is diagnostic. Anti parietal cell antibody titre may be done to identify patients of autoimmune gastritis and pernicious anaemia who are deficient in intrinsic factor, essential for absorption of vitamin B12 [5].

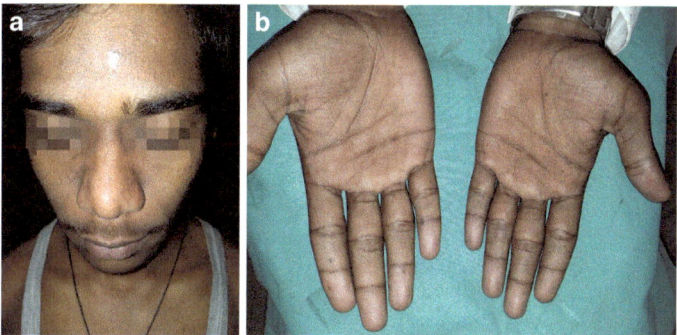

FIGURE 13.4 (**a**) Resolution of facial pigmentation after vitamin B12 supplementation. (**b**) Resolution of pigmentation of palms after vitamin B12 supplementation

The treatment is done by supplementing vitamin B12 and intramuscular injections in the form of cyanocobalamin 1000 μg is given daily for first week followed by weekly injections for next month and then monthly thereafter (Fig. 13.4a, b). Instead of injections, daily dose of Vitamin B12 1000 μg is sufficient for maintaining a normal reserve [8]. The cause of vitamin B12 should be searched for and needs to be taken care of. Strict vegetarians and patients with intrinsic factors deficiency may require lifelong prophylactic supplementation. Dual supplementation along with folate can be beneficial as clinically it is difficult to differentiate the two conditions including the neurological manifestations if laboratory testing is not possible [9].

Key Points
- Vitamin B12 deficiency may result from malabsorption or inadequate intake. The latter is almost exclusively seen in vegetarians.
- Vitamin B12 deficiency may present with isolated cutaneous and mucosal hypermelanosis. Also, affected patients may develop various systemic manifestations along with or without mucocutaneous features.

- Vitamin B12 deficiency should always be considered in the differential for diffuse hyperpigmentation of skin.
- The diagnosis is confirmed by vitamin B12 estimation and the condition is treated by parenteral or oral vitamin B12 supplementation.

References

1. Hoffbrand AV. Megaloblastic anemias. In: Fauci AS, Braunwald E, Kasper DL, et al., editors. Harrison's principles of internal medicine. 17th ed. New York: McGraw-Hill; 2008. p. 643–51.
2. Bernard M, Babior H, Franklin B. Megaloblastic anemias. In: Kasper DL, Braunwald E, Fauci AS, Hauser SL, Longo DL, Jameson JL, editors. Harrison's principles of internal medicine. 16th ed. New York: McGraw-Hill; 2005. p. 601–7.
3. Agrawala RK, Sahoo SK, Choudhury AK, Mohanty BK, Baliarsinha AK. Pigmentation in vitamin B12 deficiency masquerading Addison's pigmentation: a rare presentation. Indian J Endocrinol Metab. 2013;17(Suppl 1):S254–6.
4. Oh R, Brown DL. Vitamin B12 deficiency. Am Fam Physician. 2003;67(5):979–86.
5. Jithendriya M, Kumaran S, IB P. Addisonian pigmentation and vitamin B12 deficiency: a case series and review of the literature. Cutis. 2013;92:94–9.
6. Arora AK, Saini SS, De D, Handa S. Reticulate pigmentation associated with vitamin B12 deficiency. Indian Dermatol Online J. 2016;7(3):215–7.
7. Wadia RS, Bandishti S, Kharche M. B12 and folate deficiency: incidence and clinical features. Neurol India. 2000;48:302.
8. Pruthi RK, Tefferi A. Pernicious anemia revisited. Mayo Clin Proc. 1994;69:144–50.
9. Kannan R, Ng MJ. Cutaneous lesions and vitamin B12 deficiency: an often-forgotten link. Can Fam Physician. 2008;54(4):529–32.

Chapter 14
A Young Boy with Generalized Hyperpigmentation

Rajesh Kumar Mandal

An 8-year-old boy presented with generalized darkening of skin of 1 year duration. His mother also complained of progressive weakness, weight loss, fatigue, poor appetite, nausea and occasional vomiting. There were two episodes of syncope also. There was no history of tuberculosis or any other systemic major illness in past. There was no history of any drug therapy preceding these complaints. He was hospitalized once for hypotension, shock and weakness. On examination, his blood pressure was 80/50 mmHg. All other vital parameters were within normal limits. On cutaneous examination, there was generalized hyperpigmentation of the skin, specially the face, hands, and palms (Fig. 14.1). The palmar creases and nail bed also showed hyperpigmentation and melanonychia was observed in a few nails (Fig. 14.2). Tongue and buccal mucosa showed patchy hyperpigmentation. Biochemical tests revealed hyponatremia (129 mmol/L) with hyperkalemia (5.5 mmol/L). 8 a.m. serum cortisol level was decreased to 46 nmol/L (range: 102–535 nmol/L). Liver and renal function tests, Thyroid stimulating hormone and blood glucose were within normal limits. Complete blood counts, RBC indices, peripheral blood smear and vitamin B12 level

R. K. Mandal (✉)
North Bengal Medical College, Darjeeling, India

© Springer Nature Switzerland AG 2020
S. Kothiwala et al. (eds.), *Clinical Cases in Disorders of Melanocytes*, Clinical Cases in Dermatology,
https://doi.org/10.1007/978-3-030-22757-9_14

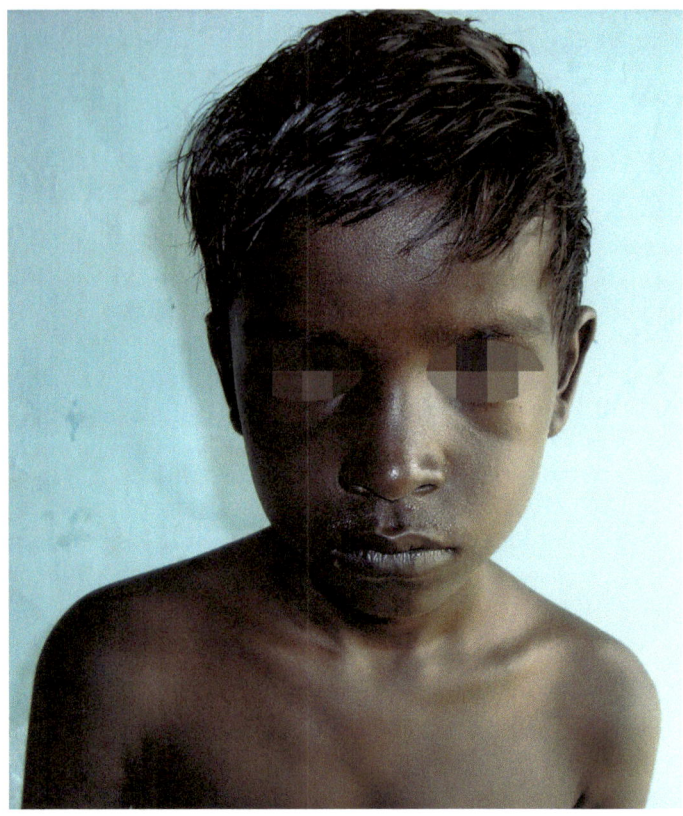

FIGURE 14.1 Generalized hyperpigmentation affecting face (Courtesy: Dr. Santoshdev P. Rathod)

estimation did not reveal any abnormality. What is your diagnosis?

1. Lichen Planus Pigmentosus
2. Addison's disease
3. Vitamin B12 deficiency
4. Nelson syndrome

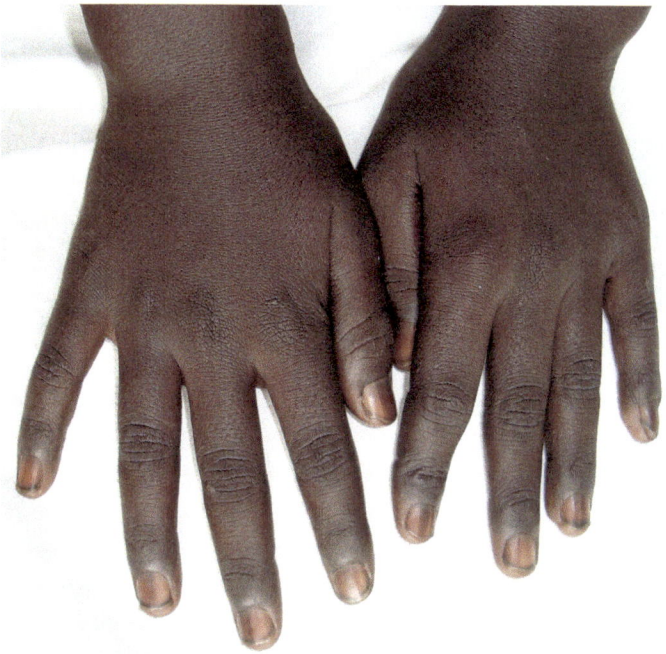

FIGURE 14.2 Hyperpigmentation of hands with nail pigmentation and melanonychia (Courtesy: Dr. Santoshdev P. Rathod)

Diagnosis

- Addison's disease

Discussion

Addison's disease is rare endocrinal disease of adrenal insufficiency. Though the exact prevalence in Indian population is not defined but countries like Great Britain where data is present shows a prevalence of 39 cases per one million population. Addison's disease is characterized by various systemic and mucocutaneous manifestations. The disease symptoms progress slowly and may become fatal with an event of illness or accident. Cutaneous and mucosal hyperpigmentation is commonly associated with Addison's disease.

Addison's disease can affect both male and females equally and can occur at any age. It was first described by Thomas Addison in year 1855 [1]. Autoimmune destruction of the adrenal gland is the main cause of this disease although Tuberculosis is also a major contributor to its cause in developing country. Among other causes fungal infection, haemochromatosis, primary or metastatic neoplasm, traumatic, iatrogenic and systemic amyloidosis are of importance [2]. As a result there is decreased secretion of cortisol which causes increased secretion of ACTH and MSH from pituitary gland. Increased MSH stimulates the melanocytes which in turn produce more melanin pigment leading to hyperpigmentation of skin [3].

The clinical symptoms start slowly which comprises chronic fatigue, decreased appetite, nausea, vomiting, generalized weakness and weight loss. The skin becomes hyperpigmented. The sun exposed skin and the bony prominences like elbows, knees and palmer creases show more prominent hyperpigmentation. As the disease progresses the mucous membrane also become hyperpigmented. The gingival, vermilion border of lip, palate, tongue and buccal mucosa all become pigmented. Nails may show longitudinal hyperpigmented lines known as melanonychia. Cutaneous hyperpigmentation is considered as hallmark of Addison's disease and is seen in most of the cases [3]. The symptoms if ignored may lead to Addisonian crisis precipitated by any event of illness or accident which is characterized by severe pain in lower back, abdomen and legs associated with severe diarrhea, vomiting leading to dehydration, low blood pressure and syncope [4].

Important differential diagnoses for Addison's disease are Vitamin B12 deficiency, Nelson syndrome, Lichen planus pigmentosus and Erythema dyschromicum perstans. Vitamin B12 deficiency is characterized by asymptomatic hyperpigmentation of extremities especially affecting dorsum of hands and feet. There may be accentuation of pigmentation over interphalangeal joints and terminal phalanges. Oral mucosal hyperpigmentation may be associated. Other features of vitamin B12 deficiency like angular stomatitis, glossitis and hair changes may also be present. Serum vitamin B12 level is diagnostic. Nelson syndrome is a pituitary tumor after adrenalectomy and is characterized by abnormal ACTH hormone secretion leading to hyperpigmentation of skin, headache, visual field abnormalities and menopause in females. Imaging studies such as Computed tomography (CT) scan and magnetic resonance imaging (MRI), and biochemical tests reveals the diagnosis. Lichen Planus Pigmentosus is a macular variety of Lichen Planus mostly seen in middle aged dark skinned individuals. It is characterized by slate grey to brown black pigmented macules which may coalesce. The pigmentation is diffuse, reticulate, perifollicular or blotchy. The cutaneous pigmentation is usually symmetrical and mucosae are spared. There are no associated systemic symptoms [3].

The plan of investigation includes confirmation of Addison's disease followed tests to find the etiology. Serum cortisol level from 8 a.m. blood sample should be performed. Serum cortisol below 83 nmol/L confirms Addison's disease. Serum electrolytes should be done and may show hyponatremia, low chloride and hyperkalemia due to absence of aldosterone which supports the diagnosis. The hypothalamic-pituitary-adrenal (HPA) axis evaluation is done by corticotrophin stimulation test, insulin tolerance test and metyrapone test [5]. Tuberculosis screening tests, search for 21-hydroxylase autoantibodies, and 17-hydroxyprogesterone estimation (for congenital adrenal hyperplasia) may be done when indicated. Imaging studies like Computed tomography (CT) scan and magnetic resonance imaging (MRI) are done to look at the size and shape of the adrenal glands and the pituitary. The adrenal glands may be enlarged with infections and cancers, but with autoimmune diseases and secondary adrenal insufficiency, the adrenal glands are often normal or small [6].

Treatment includes adequate replacement of glucocorticoids and/or mineralocorticoids. Secondary adrenal insufficiency due to hypothalamic or pituitary diseases is treated in a similar manner. An adrenal crisis is an avoidable, life-threatening complication and is treated with intravenous injections of glucocorticoids (hydrocortisone), along with correction of hypovolemia and hyponatremia by large volumes of intravenous saline solution with the sugar dextrose [5].

Key Points

- Adrenal insufficiency of Addison's disease may result from adrenal grand damage by a variety of conditions including autoimmune diseases, tuberculosis, and iatrogenic causes (sudden withdrawal following long term corticosteroid use). Sometimes, it may develop secondary to damage to hypothalamic or pituitary gland.
- The cutaneous hallmark is generalized hyperpigmentation of the skin, mucosa and nails. Systemic manifestations result from hyponatremia, hyperkalemia, and low blood glucose.
- Low cortisol level from morning (8 a.m.) sample confirms the diagnosis of Addison's disease. Further investigations are done to establish the etiology.
- Treatment is by replacement of glucocorticoids and/or mineralocorticoids. Prevention, and early treatment of adrenal crisis are essential component of management of Addison's disease.

References

1. Grossman AB. Thomas Addison and his disease. Grand Rounds. 2004;4:L8–9.
2. Stewart PM, Krone NP. The adrenal cortex. In: Kronenburg HM, Melmed S, Polonsky KS, Reed Larson P, editors. Williams textbook of endocrinology. 12th ed. Philadelphia: Saunders/Elsevier; 2011. p. 515–20.

3. Ten S, New M, Maclaren N. Clinical review 130: Addison's disease 2001. J Clin Endocrinol Metab. 2001;86:2909–22.
4. O'Connell S, Siafarikas A. Addison disease—diagnosis and initial management. Aust Fam Physician. 2010;39:834–7.
5. Michels A, Michels N. Addison disease: early detection and treatment principles. Am Fam Physician. 2014;89(7):563–8.
6. Brandão Neto RA, de Carvalho JF. Diagnosis and classification of Addison's disease (autoimmune adrenalitis). Autoimmun Rev. 2014;13(4–5):408–11.

Part IV
Hypomelanotic Disorders

Chapter 15
A Girl with Hypopigmented Patch on Cheek

Pooja Nupur

A 6-year-old girl was brought to the outpatient department with complaints of an asymptomatic white coloured irregular lesion of the left cheek (Fig. 15.1). Mother observed the lesion 3 years back and gave the history of treatment for vitiligo for three months from a general practitioner with no relief. Mother gave the history of slight increase in size of lesion with age. There was no history of any skin disease or any injury prior to development of lesion. Rest of the history was non-contributory. On examination, patient had solitary hypopigmented patch with irregular, but well-defined, border on cheek. On diascopy, the margin of the lesion did not fade (Fig. 15.2). Based on the case description and photograph, what is your diagnosis?

1. Nevus depigmentosus
2. Hypomelanosis of Ito
3. Nevus Anaemicus
4. Piebaldism

P. Nupur (✉)
Nalanda Medical College and Hospital, Patna, India

© Springer Nature Switzerland AG 2020
S. Kothiwala et al. (eds.), *Clinical Cases in Disorders of Melanocytes*, Clinical Cases in Dermatology,
https://doi.org/10.1007/978-3-030-22757-9_15

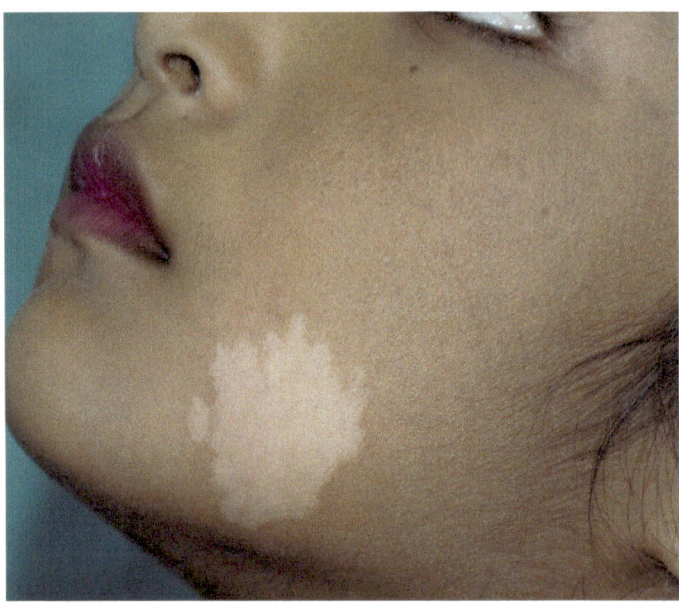

FIGURE 15.1 Well demarcated hypopigmented patch on cheek. Note serrated margin

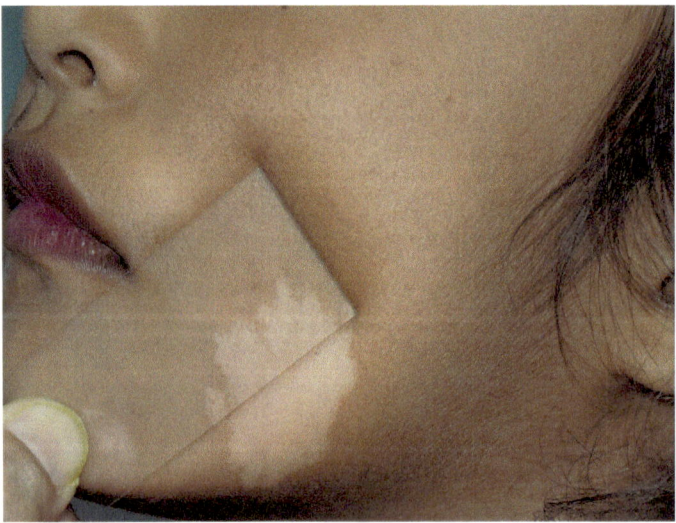

FIGURE 15.2 The margins are not fading or disappearing on diascopy

Diagnosis

- Nevus depigmentosus

Discussion

Nevus depigmentosus (ND), also known as nevus achro-micus, is a rare congenital non-progressive hypopigmented nevus. It can affect any race or gender. Exact cause of nevus depigmentosus is still not clearly understood. It is believed to be a cutaneous pigmentary mosaic disorder wherein functional defect of melanocytes with morphological abnormalities of melanosomes are major factors resulting in ND. Melanocytes have reduced ability to produce melanin and to transfer melanosomes to keratinocytes. Melanosomes can be diminished in number, heteromorphic, aggregated in melanocytes, or located in membrane bound aggregates [1]. It presents with solitary well circumscribed hypo- to depigmented patch, with an irregular serrated but well defined border, which do not cross midline. Many times smaller lesions may appear distributed over edge giving it a splashed paint appearance. It is commonly visible at birth and may appear later in adulthood. Commonly affected sites are trunk, neck, face and proximal part of extremities but it may occur at anywhere on the body. It may increases in size with the growth of the body and after reaching its maximum dimensions it usually remains unchanged throughout life. In contrast to what its name suggests, the nevus depigmentosus presents itself as a hypopigmentation rather than a depigmentation [2]. Three clinical subtypes have been described:

1. Isolated or localised form (solitary and well defined lesion)—It is most common pattern.
2. Segmental form (unilateral, band shaped sometimes Blaschkoid distribution)
3. Systematized form (extensive whorls or linear streaks of hypopigmentation, following lines of Blaschko): This subtype is very rare and may have extra cutaneous manifestations such as seizures, mental retardation, hemi hypertrophy,

and yellow hair and may have been categorised as hypomelanosis of Ito [1].

The diagnosis is usually made clinically. Coupe et al., in 1976, have proposed a diagnostic criteria and diagnosis of ND is made when [2]

- Leukoderma is present at birth or of early onset
- No alteration in the distribution of leukoderma throughout life
- No alteration in texture or change in sensation in the affected area
- Absence of hyperpigmented border

Histological studies on lesional skin compared with perilesional normal skin shows a marked reduction in melanin, with normal to reduced number of melanocytes with S-100 stain and less reactivity with 3,4-dihydroxyphenylalanine reaction. There is no pigment incontinence. On electron microscopy melanocytes show stubby dendrites and autophagosomes with aggregates of melanosomes. Diascopy test is negative in ND and positive in its close differential nevus anemicus [1]. Dermoscopy shows off-white color in ND which helps it in differentiating from vitiligo (chalky white color). Other findings include faint pigment network over the lesion, and serrated borders extending onto the normal skin as "pseudopods" (Fig. 15.3) [3].

The common clinical differential diagnoses include nevus anemicus, piebaldism and hypomelanosis of Ito. Nevus anemicus is an uncommon hypopigmented disorder which results from vasoconstriction of small vessels due to increased sensitivity of adrenergic receptor of the endothelial cells of the affected area. It is usually present at birth as hypopigmented macule of variable size. Borders merge with surrounding skin on applying pressure. It can be illustrated by putting glass slide with pressure known as diascopy test. It becomes more visible on emotional stress. Rarely, it may be associated with port-wine stain and neurofibromatosis type 1 [4]. Piebaldism is a rare autosomal dominant condition with

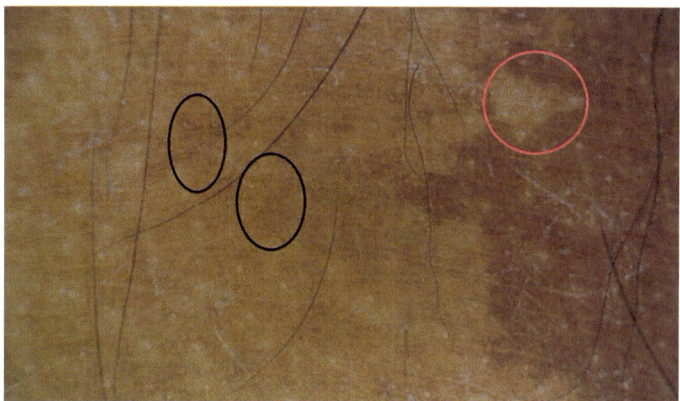

Figure 15.3 Dermoscopy of the lesion shows faint, but normal reticular pattern of pigment within the depigmented area (black circles), and pseudopods (red circle) (Courtesy: Dr. Shekhar Neema)

mutation in the c-kit proto-oncogene, mapped to the proximal long arm of chromosome 4 or deletions in the SLUG gene, which is zinc-finger neural crest transcription factor. It is present at birth with extensive, symmetrically distributed depigmented macules mainly on forehead (often triangular in shape), front of thorax and extremities. The depigmented patch is often associated with hyperpigmented macules within areas of depigmentation. The white forelock is present in 80–90% of affected individuals. Eyebrow and eyelash hair may also be affected. It is may be associated with Waardenburg's syndrome—a syndrome of White forelock, Heterochromia iridis, and Deafmutism among other features [5]. Hypomelanosis of Ito (HOI) is rare genetic sporadic disease with autosomal dominant, recessive and X linked inheritance. HOI and ND can be considered phenotypic expression of mosaicism in pigment gene. Clinically it present similar to systematized pattern of ND in which hypopigmented areas consisting of bilateral or unilateral whorls and streaks corresponding to the lines of Blaschko. Other types of pigmentary pattern are possible checkerboard pattern, phylloid pattern, and patchy pattern without midline separation. It is likely that mutations in pigmentary gene occur much earlier in HOI and thus more body structures are involved (62–94% chance of systemic involvement). The heterogeneity of genetic anomalies may be due to the presence of multiple loci coding for pigment related proteins. Common systemic involvement is neurological (epilepsy, developmental delay, microcephaly, hypotonia, hyperkinesias, deafness), skeletal (scoliosis, hypertelorism, coarse facies, nose and ear abnormalities, syndactyly, polydactyly) and ocular (ptosis, microphthalmia, nystagmus, strabismus). The distinction between whorled ND and HOI is unclear at times. Cases of HOI without extra cutaneous anomalies have often been categorized as ND, whereas cases of ND associated with extra cutaneous anomalies may have been categorized as HOI [6]. Other clinical differentials include ash leaf macule, Hansen's disease and pityriasis alba [2].

Usually ND doesn't require any active treatment. While thorough and gentle counselling is often sufficient, various treatment modalities include Camouflage, surgical grafting and excimer laser may be tried for cosmetic reasons [7].

Key Points

- Nevus depigmentosus is uncommon congenital pigmentary disorder which may cause significant psychological morbidity in patients with skin of color.
- Clinically, nevus depigmentosus is characterized by a hypopigmented patch with serrated border. The lesion grows in size in proportion to the growth of the body and eventually becomes stable.
- Detailed clinical examination and investigations may be required to rule out systemic involvement in patients with extensive lesions.
- Usually counselling about the nature of disease is required. Some patients may seek treatment for aesthetic reasons.

References

1. Deb S, Sarkar R, Samanta AB. A brief review of nevus depigmentosus. Pigment Int. 2014;1:56–8.
2. Ullah F, Schwartz RA. Review of a mark of distinction. Int J Dermatol. 2019. https://doi.org/10.1111/ijd.14393.
3. Ankad BS, Shah S. Dermoscopy of nevus depigmentosus. Pigment Int. 2017;4:121–3.
4. Salvini C, Fabroni C, Francalanci S, Massi D, Difonzo EM. Generalized nevus anaemicus in an adult. J Eur Acad Dermatol Venereol. 2007;21(8):1142–4.
5. Agarwal S, Ojha A. Piebaldism: a brief report and review of the literature. Indian Dermatol Online J. 2012;3(2):144–7.
6. Ream M. Hypomelanosis of Ito. Handb Clin Neurol. 2015;132:281–9.
7. Mulekar SV, Issa AA, Aisa AA. Nevus depigmentosus treated by melanocyte–keratinocyte transplantation. J Cutan Aesthet Surg. 2011;4(1):29–32.

Chapter 16
Congenital Absence of Pigmentation in Skin and Hair with Diminished Vision

Gunjan Jha

A 6-year-old boy, born out of a consanguineous marriage presented with white skin and hair, photophobia and diminished vision. The onset was congenital. There was complete lack of pigment in the skin, hair, eyebrows and eyelashes (Fig. 16.1). The family history was absent. Ophthalmologic examination revealed bluish translucent iris, nystagmus, reduced visual acuity (1/10) and foveal hypoplasia. He had normal physical and mental development. His routine laboratory parameters (including peripheral blood smear) were within normal limits. No other congenital or systemic abnormalities was found. Based on the clinical details and physical examination, what is the diagnosis?

1. Chediak-Higashi syndrome
2. Cross Syndrome
3. Oculocutaneous albinism
4. Hermansky-Pudlak syndrome

G. Jha (✉)
Department of Internal Medicine, Fortis Hospital, Noida, India

© Springer Nature Switzerland AG 2020
S. Kothiwala et al. (eds.), *Clinical Cases in Disorders of Melanocytes*, Clinical Cases in Dermatology,
https://doi.org/10.1007/978-3-030-22757-9_16

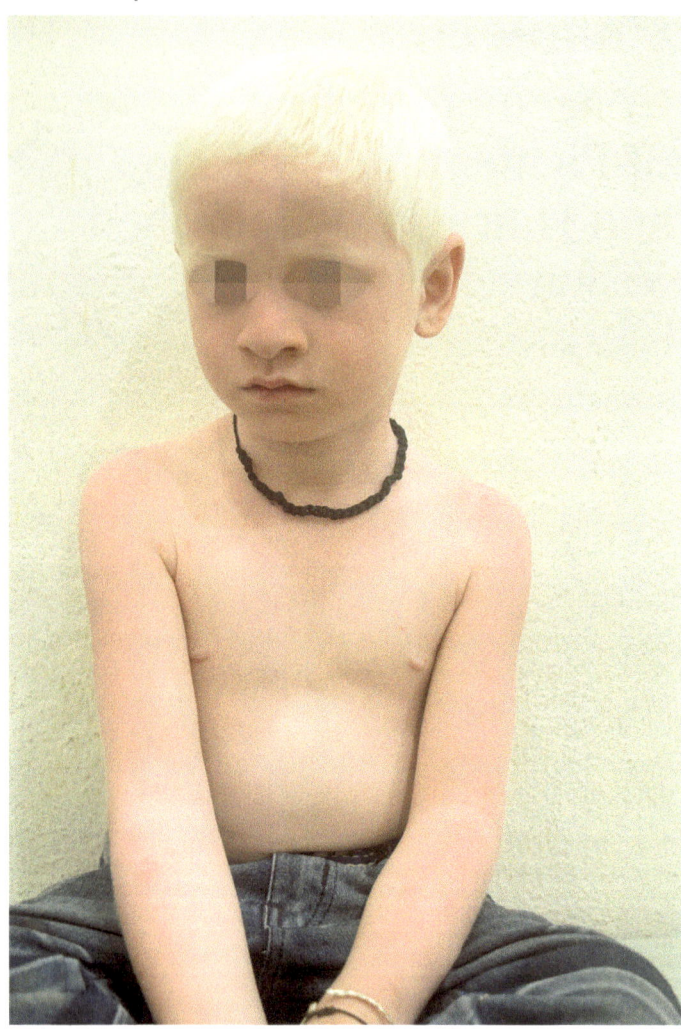

FIGURE 16.1 Generalized loss of pigmentation of skin and hair. (Courtesy: Dr. Piyush Kumar)

Diagnosis

• Oculocutaneous albinism

Discussion

Oculocutaneous albinism (OCA) is the most common inherited, heterogeneous disorder of generalized hypopigmentation involving skin, hair and eyes. It has five forms: OCA1A, OCA1B (yellow albinism), OCA2 (brown albinism), OCA3 (rufous/red type) and OCA4 (least common) [1]. The global estimated frequency of OCA is 1:20000. The major two forms, OCA1 (tyrosine-negative) and OCA2 (tyrosine-positive) constitute 90% of the cases seen worldwide and OCA2 is the most prevalent form [2]. OCA3 and OCA4 are rare.

In OCA1A, genetic mutations in TYR gene completely abolish tyrosinase activity, while mutations rendering some enzyme activity result in OCA1B allowing some accumulation of melanin pigment over time. The gene implicated in OCA2 is P, important for normal processing and transport of melanosomal proteins such as TYR and TYRP1. Mutations in Tyrp1 gene in OCA3 result in delayed maturation and an early degradation of Tyr. Mutations in the membrane-associated transporter protein gene (MATP) cause OCA4 [1].

OCA1A is the most severe type showing complete absence of melanin production throughout life. The skin, hair, eyelashes and eyebrows are all white, and skin does not tan. Iris are light blue to pink and completely translucent along with intense photophobia and visual acuity 1/10 or less. The prominent ocular anomalies include congenital nystagmus, reduced pigmentation of the retinal pigment epithelium, foveal hypoplasia, misrouting of the optic nerve fibres at optic chiasma resulting in strabismus and reduced stereoscopic vision [2]. In OCA1B, OCA2 and OCA4, the hair and skin may develop some pigment with time, irises are green/

brown and visual acuity improves. OCA3 patients have red hair and reddish brown skin with no detectable visual anomalies are not always detectable [1]. A few other unusual ocular changes are Duane retraction syndrome, corneal mesodermal dysgenesis, and congenital glaucoma. Risk of development of non-melanoma skin cancer is also high in OCA [3].

Chediak–Higashi syndrome (CHS) is a rare, autosomal recessive multi-system disorder caused by mutation in LYST gene. It is characterized by hypopigmentation of the skin, eyes and hair, prolonged bleeding time, easy bruisability, recurrent infection, abnormal NK cell function and peripheral neuropathy [4]. Most of the patients develop an accelerated phase of the disease characterized by fever, jaundice, hepatosplenomegaly, lymphadenopathy, pancytopenia, coagulopathy and neurological abnormalities, unlike in OCA. The presence of massive peroxidase-positive lysosomal inclusion in the leukocytes, fibroblasts and melanocytes is diagnostic [4].

Hermansky-Pudlak syndrome is a rare autosomal recessive disorder characterized by reduced pigmentation of skin, hair, iris and retina, platelet storage-pool deficiency and lysosomal accumulation of ceroid lipofuscin in various tissues including reticuloendothelial system. It mostly results from the mutation in HPS 1 and 3 genes associated with the formation of lysosome-related organelles. Although oculocutaneous presentation simulate the picture of OCA but the systemic findings such as bleeding diathesis, interstitial lung fibrosis, granulomatous colitis, cardiomyopathy and renal dysfunction help to differentiate it from OCA [5].

Cross syndrome or Cross-McKusick-Breen Syndrome is an inherited (autosomal recessive) oculocerebral syndrome, characterized by hypopigmentation of the skin and hair, and oculocerebral abnormalities. The common features shared with OCA include autosomal recessive trait, unusually light skin color, silvery-gray hair, hypopigmented iris and nystagmus [6]. There are certain other characteristic findings which are frequently present in this syndrome. These are delayed developmental milestones (psychomotor retardation), corneal opacities, microphthalmia, iris atrophy, cataract, optic nerve atrophy, gingival fibromatosis, high arched palate, oligophrenia, dolichocephaly, athetosis, spastic paraplegia and Dandy-Walker type cystic malformation of posterior fossa [6].

Genetic counseling and prenatal diagnosis is an integral part of management of OCA. The gene mutational analysis is done by denaturing high performance liquid chromatography and single stranded conformational polymorphism followed by DNA sequencing.

Treatment is given according to the types and severity of OCA. Bifocal glasses help to correct low visual acuity and dark/photochromic lenses are used to prevent photophobia. Surgery of the ocular muscles may be done to cure nystagmus. For strabismus, it may be necessary to patch one eye in children to force the non-preferred eye to be used. Most people with severe forms of OCA do not tan and easily get sunburned, therefore sunscreens are recommended with at least a sun protection factor of 15.

Key Points
- OCA is the most common inherited disorder of generalized hypopigmentation due to genetic defects in melanin biosynthesis.
- It has five forms: OCA1A, OCA1B, OCA2, OCA3 and OCA4.
- OCA2 is the most common type and affects 1:4000 of the population in some parts of Africa.
- OCA1A is most severe type with complete lack of pigmentation in skin, hair and eyes. There is no pigment synthesis with age.
- Other types are milder and develop pigmentation over time.
- Hematologic tests, ophthalmic and systemic examination are mandatory to rule out other syndromic entities presenting with partial OCA.

References

1. Grønskov K, Ek J, Brondum-Nielsen K. Oculocutaneous albinism. Orphanet J Rare Dis. 2007;2:43.
2. Rao VA, Swathi P, Chaitra, Thappa DM. Bilateral keratoconus with oculocutaneous albinism. Indian J Dermatol Venereol Leprol. 2008;74:407–9.
3. Jethani J, Parija S, Shetty S, Vijayalakshmi P. Duane retraction syndrome associated with oculocutaneous albinism: an ocular miswiring. Indian J Ophthalmol. 2006;54:283–4.
4. Rudramurthy P, Lokanatha H. Chediak-Higashi syndrome: a case series from Karnataka, India. Indian J Dermatol. 2015;60:524.
5. Bagheri A, Abdollahi A. Hermansky-pudlak syndrome; a case report. J Ophthalmic Vis Res. 2010;5(4):269–72.
6. Tezcan I, Demir E, Asan E, Kale G, Mitftitoglu SF, Kotiloglu E. A new case of oculocerebral hypopigmentation syndrome (Cross syndrome) with additional findings. Clin Genet. 1997;51:118–21.

Chapter 17
Slowly Progressive Depigmented Macules on Face and Hands in a Child

Anup Kumar Tiwary

A 11-year-old child presented to our outpatient department with slowly progressive depigmented patches on face for past 2 years. On examination, loss of pigmentation was noted on forehead, periocular region, bridge of nose, and lips. White hairs of right eyebrow were also noted. Lesions were asymptomatic and non-scaly (Fig. 17.1). There was no history of pre-existing dermatosis or chemical application at the site. Her routine laboratory parameters including thyroid profile were within normal limits. Her mother has similar lesions on her hands. Based on the case description and the photograph, what is your diagnosis?

1. Chemical leukoderma
2. Idiopathic guttate hypomelanosis
3. Vitiligo
4. Pityriasis versicolor

A. K. Tiwary (✉)
Department of Dermatology, Subharti Medical College,
Meerut, Uttar Pradesh, India

© Springer Nature Switzerland AG 2020   135
S. Kothiwala et al. (eds.), *Clinical Cases in Disorders
of Melanocytes*, Clinical Cases in Dermatology,
https://doi.org/10.1007/978-3-030-22757-9_17

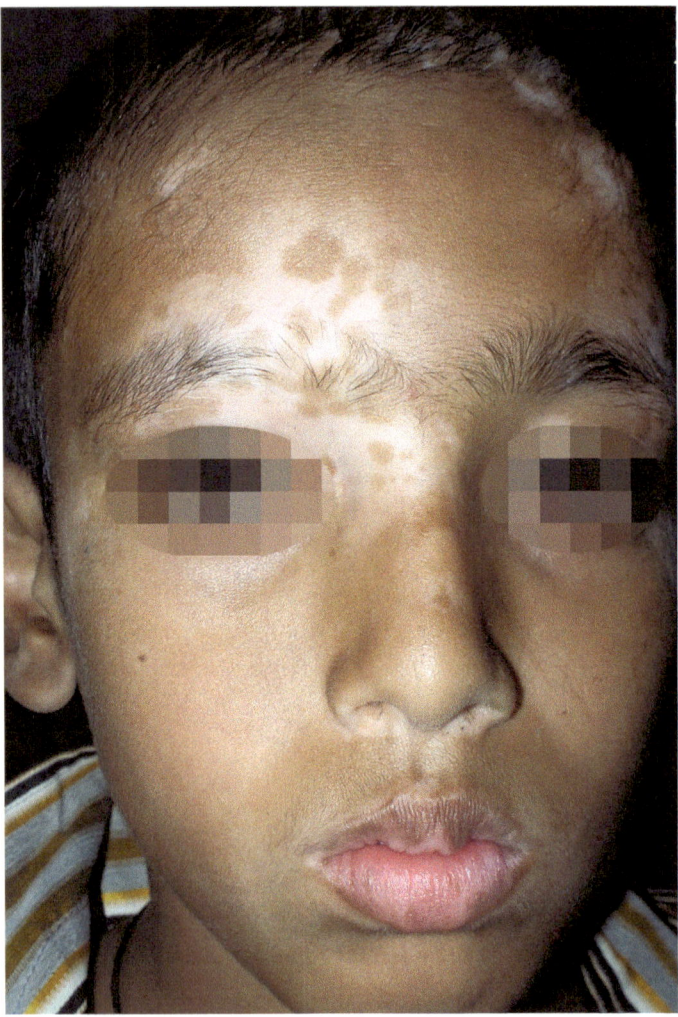

FIGURE 17.1 Depigmented macules on face predominantly involving forehead, nose, periocular area and lips (Courtesy: Dr. Piyush Kumar)

Diagnosis

• Vitiligo

Discussion

Vitiligo is an acquired autoimmune, depigmentary disorder due to destruction of melanocytes, characterized by depigmented macules affecting the skin and/or mucous membranes with variable progression and intermittent remission [1]. The loss of melanocytes may also be evident in the eyes, hair bulbs and ears, leading to alterations in both structure and function of these organs. It can occur at any age, but it usually occurs before the age of 20 years in nearly 50% of patients and affects nearly 1–2% of the world population [2]. With polygenic inheritance with variable penetrance, positive family history ranges from 6 to 40%. Triggering factors may be emotional stress, drug intake, infections, trauma (Koebner's phenomenon). Being of autoimmune in origin, it has been seen to be associated with other autoimmune disorders and endocrine disorders mostly of thyroid [1].

The pathogenesis of melanocyte destruction in vitiligo is complex and yet to know much about. There are many proposed theories such as an intrinsic defect of melanocytes and autoimmune destruction, cytotoxicity, neural theory, oxidant-antioxidant mechanisms and melanocytorrhagy. It is being widely accepted that there may be different pathomechanisms for different subtypes of vitiligo [2].

Vitiligo has been classified in many ways and various types. Conventionally, there are four types: generalized or vitiligo vulgaris (most common), acrofacial, segmental, and universal [2]. It typically presents with asymptomatic, well-demarcated, chalky-white or ivory-white, round or oval macules with scalloped margins [2]. The margin may be hyperpigmented. Due to the presence of multiple shades, some morphological variants have been described such as trichrome, quadrichrome and pentachrome vitiligo [2]. The presence of leukotrichia indicates poor prognosis. Histopathology reveals complete absence of melanocytes, increased numbers of Langerhans cells in epidermis and lymphocytic infiltrates and/or spongiotic foci at the edge of the active vitiligo lesions.

Chemical leukoderma is an acquired condition of loss of skin pigmentation resulting from repeated exposure to a chemical agent. Phenols and catechols as well as sulfhydryl compounds are most common culprits [3]. The contact site with the chemical and even non-contact areas may also develop depigmented patches. Confetti-like macules are another characteristic feature. The sign of contact dermatitis may be seen but in minority of cases. Histopathology is not specific although lichenoid mononuclear dermal infiltrates are more common and Langerhans cells are normal in numbers [3]. Avoidance of the causative agent may lead to spontaneous repigmentation.

Pityriasis versicolor is a superficial mycosis caused by lipophilic yeast, Malassezia furfur. It is clinically characterized by the presence of hypopigmented or reddish-brown macular patches with fine/furfuraceous scales over neck, upper trunk and shoulder. Potassium hydroxide (KOH) testing of skin scraping demonstrates "spaghetti and meatballs" appearance due to the presence of spores and hypha [4]. On Wood's lamp, it gives yellowish-white or copper-orange fluorescence.

Idiopathic guttate hypomelanosis is a common acquired disorder, usually occurring after fourth decade of life. The commonest sites are shin and extensor of forearm and face and trunk are usually spared. The classical individual lesions are small (2–5 mm in diameter), very sharply defined hypopigmented macules, usually numbering between 10 and 30, but numerous lesions may occur [4]. On histopathology, there is epidermal atrophy with flattened rete ridges and reduced numbers of hypoactive melanocytes.

There are various treatment modalities for vitiligo. They are topical/intralesional/oral steroids, immunomodulators, other immunosuppressives, PUVA (oral/topical), PUVASOL (PUVA using natural sunlight), UVB, narrow-band UVB, 308-nm excimer laser and skin grafting surgeries [1].

Key Points

- Vitiligo is an acquired depigmentary disorder due to auto-immune destruction of epidermal melanocytes.
- Koebnerization is the specific feature.
- Other autoimmune disorders especially hypothyroidism should be ruled out in all cases.
- Histopathologic hallmarks include complete absence of melanocytes and Langerhans cells in epidermis.

References

1. Parsad D. Vitiligo: emerging paradigms. Indian J Dermatol Venereol Leprol. 2012;78:17–8.
2. Sehgal VN, Srivastava G. Vitiligo: compendium of clinico-epidemiological features. Indian J Dermatol Venereol Leprol. 2007;73:149–56.
3. Bonamonte D, Vestita M, Romita P, Filoni A, Foti C, Angelini G. Chemical leukoderma. Dermatitis. 2016;27(3):90–9.
4. Patel AB, Kubba R, Kubba A. Clinicopathological correlation of acquired hypopigmentary disorders. Indian J Dermatol Venereol Leprol. 2013;79:376–82.

Chapter 18
Loss of Skin Pigmentation on Feet in a Female

Anup Kumar Tiwary

A 35-year-old female came to our outpatient department presenting with depigmented patches over dorsum of feet. Few months back, she noticed loss of pigmentation on both feet. She denied any pre-existing dermatosis or traumatic injury at the site. There was no cutaneous or systemic complaint. No such personal or family history was present. On cutaneous examination, the lesions were sharply defined, depigmented macules on dorsum of both feet confined to the site in contact with the strap of slipper (made up of rubber). There were no scaling, atrophy or scarring except some erythema (Fig. 18.1). Routine laboratory parameters were within normal limits and systemic investigations were non-contributory. Based on the history, clinical description and photographs, what is your diagnosis?

1. Vitiligo
2. Chemical leukoderma
3. Nevus depigmentosus
4. Discoid lupus erythematosus

A. K. Tiwary (✉)
Department of Dermatology, Subharti Medical College, Meerut, Uttar Pradesh, India

© Springer Nature Switzerland AG 2020   141
S. Kothiwala et al. (eds.), *Clinical Cases in Disorders of Melanocytes*, Clinical Cases in Dermatology, https://doi.org/10.1007/978-3-030-22757-9_18

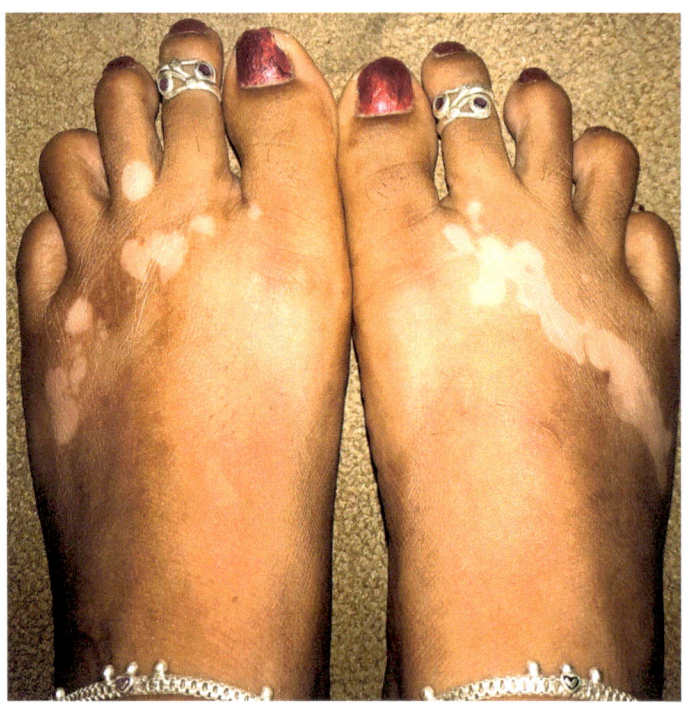

FIGURE 18.1 Sharply defined, depigmented macules on dorsum of feet confined to the site in contact with the strap of slipper ('v' shaped configuration) (Courtesy: Dr. Sunil K. Kothiwala)

Diagnosis

- Chemical leukoderma

Discussion

Chemical leukoderma is an acquired cause of loss of skin pigmentation induced by repeated, cutaneous exposure to specific melanocytotoxic chemical agents [1]. Ingestion and inhalation may also lead to this condition. Such agents can be occupational (industrial chemicals) or non-occupational (household products) [1]. The most common culprits are aromatic and aliphatic derivatives of phenols and catechol, and sulfhydryl compounds. Monobenzylether of hydroquinone (MBEH) is the first identified chemical to cause leukoderma. Other such agents are mercurial, arsenic, benzoyl peroxide, tretinoin, cinnamic aldehyde, paraphenylene diamine (PPD, in hair dye and rubber gloves) and many more [1]. In genetically susceptible persons, such chemicals, on repeated applications, can lead to the loss of pigmentation at the site of contact and sometimes, at remote site [2].

The pathogenesis of chemical leukoderma is different from vitiligo. It includes TRAIL (tumor necrosis factor related apoptosis-inducing ligands) induced apoptosis of melanocytes, inhibition of melanogenesis by blocking tyrosinase by phenolic compounds (structurally similar to tyrosine) and oxidative damage to melanocytes mediated by tyrosinase-related protein-1(Tyrp1) [3]. In genetically susceptible individuals, melanocytes are unable to withstand the Tyrp1 mediated oxidative stress resulting in death.

The onset delay varies from months to years depending upon the dose and frequency of the exposure. All age groups may be affected, although adults have a much higher incidence. Any body site may be affected. In occupational settings, the hands and forearms are commonly involved. In non-occupational cases, the scalp and face are often affected. The forehead, hands, and feet are affected in Indian patients owing to the use of "bindi" and "alta" [1]. Non-contact distant sites may also get involved in some cases due to autotransfer by hands or by lymphatic or hematogenous spread in case of systemic ingestion. Clinically, depigmented macules of chemical leukoderma appear similar to that seen in vitiligo. However, lesions are usually off-white in color and may not be sharply defined as seen in vitiligo [1]. Wood's lamp examination may be helpful to enhance the indistinct macules in many cases. Contact dermatitis is not a prerequisite for the development of chemical leukoderma and depigmentation is unlikely to occur in most of the cases of contact dermatitis. However in some cases, the same offending chemical may lead to contact dermatitis as well as chemical leukoderma, therefore itching may be an associated complaint. In most of the cases, numerous acquired round/oval confetti-like or pea-sized macules may also be seen [1]. The spreading pattern may also be helpful. A history of gradual coalescence of small discrete macules rather than the development of large macules with perifollicular sparing suggests chemical leukoderma. The presence of small confetti-like macules depends on the time of the clinical observation because they have a tendency to confluence. Histopathology in chemical leukoderma is not specific. It reveals lichenoid mononuclear infiltration in dermis and reduced/absent melanocytes.

Vitiligo is an acquired and autoimmune pigmentary disorder, characterized by well-demarcated, chalky-white macules with or without scalloped hyperpigmented border. Although it is not easy to reliably differentiate vitiligo from chemical leukoderma, trichrome morphology, koebnerization, leukotrichia, negative history of repeated exposure to a suspected chemical and lesional progression point in favour of vitiligo [1]. On histopathology in active lesions, increased numbers of Langerhans cells in epidermis and lymphocytes in the superficial dermis also support the diagnosis of vitiligo. A carefully done patch testing with suitable vehicles and fully informed consent may be useful to rule out vitiligo.

Nevus depigmentosus is a form of cutaneous mosaicism characterized by congenital, non-progressive cutaneous hypomelanosis due to dysfunctional melanocytes and abnormal melanosomes. It usually presents at birth as a solitary, circumscribed, hypopigmented macule with serrated border (splashed paint appearance) mostly on trunk, neck and proximal limbs. It remains unchanged throughout life after body's maximum physical growth [4].

Discoid lupus erythematosus (DLE) is a chronic form of cutaneous lupus that typically presents with depigmented scaly plaques with central atrophy and hyperpigmented rim. Central scarring is usually not seen in early lesions. The photoexposed sites are commonly involved and females are more prone due to its autoimmune origin. The characteristic histopathologic findings (follicular plugging, dermal perivascular and periadnexal lymphohistiocytic infiltrates, basal layer degeneration, apoptotic keratinocytes, thickened basement membrane) can reliably differentiate DLE from other disorders of depigmentation in case of any suspicion.

Avoidance of the causative agent may lead to spontaneous gradual repigmentation in months, but treatments commonly used in vitiligo such as narrow-band ultraviolet B (UVB) phototherapy, psoralen plus ultraviolet A (PUVA) photochemotherapy, or topical immunosuppressants, often are necessary [3].

Key Points
- Chemical leukoderma is typically localized to the site of application and may also spread to remote, unexposed locations.
- History of repeated cutaneous or systemic exposure to a chemical is present.
- Phenols and catechol derivatives are most common melanocytotoxic agents.
- Contact dermatitis is not a prerequisite for the development of chemical leukoderma.
- Confetti-like macules are characteristically present in most of the cases of leukoderma.
- Spontaneous repigmentation is evident in many cases after avoidance of the offending chemical/s.

References

1. Bonamonte D, Vestita M, Romita P, Filoni A, Foti C, Angelini G. Chemical leukoderma. Dermatitis. 2016;27(3):90–9.
2. Ghosh S, Mukhopadhyay S. Chemical leucoderma: a clinico-aetiological study of 864 cases in the perspective of a developing country. Br J Dermatol. 2009;160:40.
3. Harris JE. Chemical-induced vitiligo. Dermatol Clin. 2017;35(2):151–61.
4. Deb S, Sarkar R, Samanta AB. A brief review of nevus depigmentosus. Pigment Int. 2014;1:56–8.

Chapter 19
A Young Man with Hypopigmented Macules on Trunk and Multiple Shiny Nodules Over Face

Avijit Mondal and Subhash Dasarathan

A 19-year-old male presented to the dermatology OPD with hypopigmented skin lesions on trunk and limbs for 6 months, along with complaints of decreased sensation over both lower legs. Cutaneous examination showed bilaterally distributed multiple hypopigmented and slightly erythematous ill-defined macules, papules and plaques on upper limb and abdomen. There was multiple, soft to firm, dusky erythematous plaques and nodules on the face with similar lesions involving ear (Fig. 19.1). Similar hypopigmented macules, dull red nodules and plaques were seen on back (Fig. 19.2). Bilateral non-tender thickening of ulnar and common peroneal nerves were noted. Loss of sensation of temperature, touch, and diminished pain perception were elicited in both the lower legs along with dryness and loss of hair. There is no history of similar lesions in family members. There was no history of cough or difficulty in breathing. No generalized lymphadenopathy and no organomegaly were found.

A. Mondal (✉) · S. Dasarathan
College of Medicine and JNM Hospital, Kalyani, India

© Springer Nature Switzerland AG 2020
S. Kothiwala et al. (eds.), *Clinical Cases in Disorders of Melanocytes*, Clinical Cases in Dermatology,
https://doi.org/10.1007/978-3-030-22757-9_19

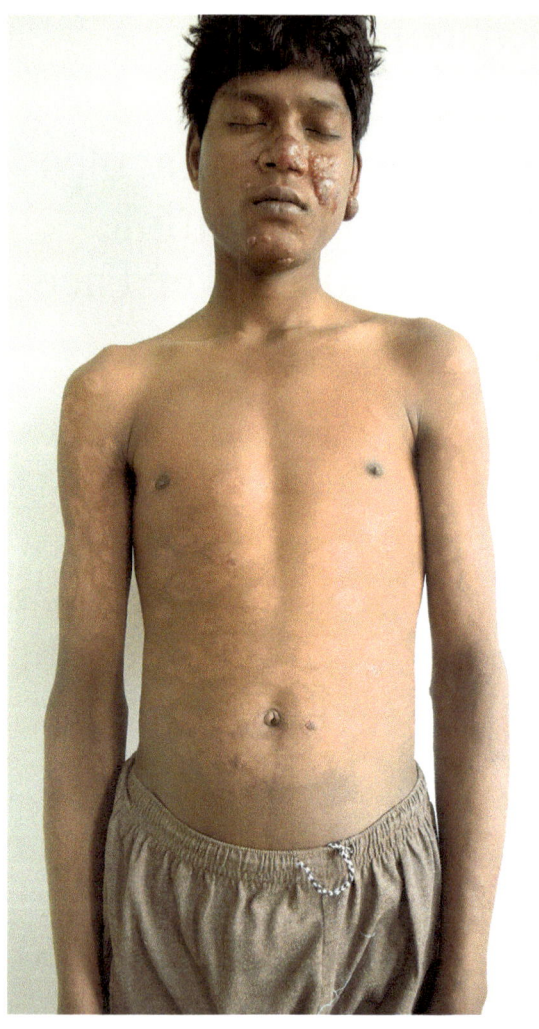

FIGURE 19.1 Multiple hypopigmented slightly erythematous macules and few papules and plaques on abdomen and right upper limb. Note plaques and nodules on face with involvement of ears (Courtesy: Dr. Piyush Kumar)

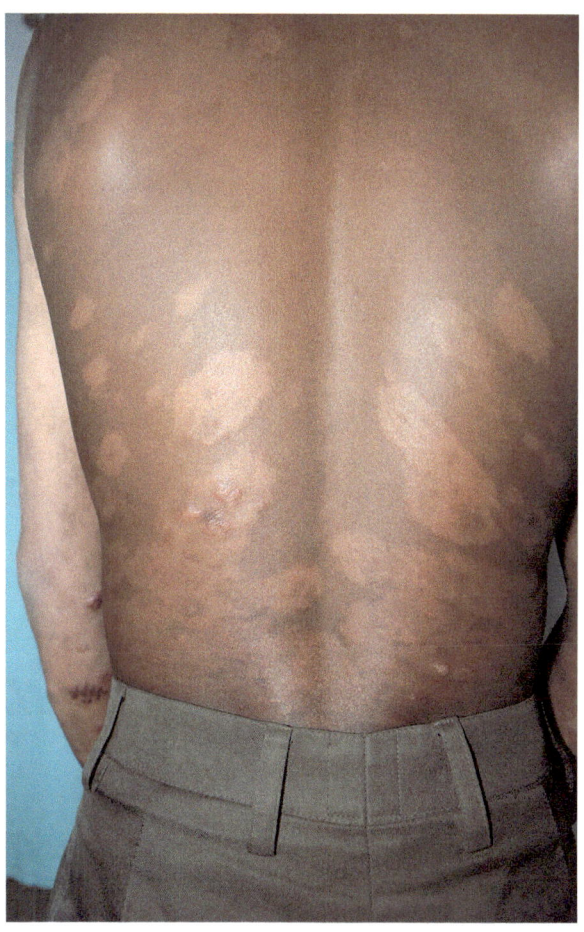

FIGURE 19.2 Multiple hypopigmented, slightly erythematous macules and few papules and plaques on the back (Courtesy: Dr. Piyush Kumar)

Based on the case description and the photographs what is your diagnosis?

1. Post Kala Azar dermal leishmaniasis
2. Lepromatous leprosy
3. Cutaneous lymphoma
4. Sarcoidosis

Diagnosis

• Lepromatous leprosy (LL)

Histopathology demonstrated flattened epidermis, dermal infiltration by foamy macrophage and few lymphocytes and a normal area (Grenz zone) in between epidermis and dermal cellular infiltrate (Fig. 19.3a). Fite Faraco stain showed numerous *M. leprae* bacilli, occurring singly and in globi (Fig. 19.3b).

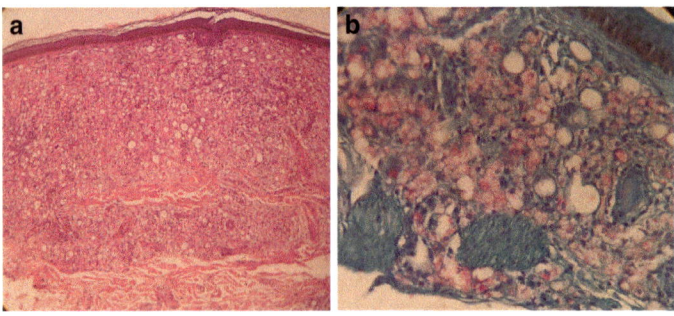

FIGURE 19.3 (**a**) Flattened epidermis, dermal macrophage infiltration and a normal area in between epidermis and dermal infiltrate (H&E, ×100) (Courtesy: Dr. Piyush Kumar). (**b**) Numerous *M. leprae* bacilli as globi (Fire Faraco staining, ×100) (Courtesy: Dr. Piyush Kumar)

Discussion

Leprosy or Hansen's disease is a chronic mildly infectious disease caused by *Mycobacterium leprae* affecting the peripheral nerves, skin and in highly bacillated state, the internal organs also. The three cardinal features of leprosy are hypopigmented or reddish skin lesions with definite loss of sensation, involvement of peripheral nerves as demonstrated by definite thickening with loss of sensation and skin smear positive for AFB (acid fast bacilli) [1]. The clinical features of leprosy depend on the bacillary multiplication and the host's cell mediated immune response.

In LL (lepromatous) type, once the bacilli enter the host, they multiply freely due to the defective cell mediated immune response and proceed to involve the nerves and skin along with other structures such as eye, reticuloendothelial system, mucous membranes, endothelium of blood vessels, involuntary muscles (dartos and arrectorpili), voluntary muscles and testes. Hypopigmentation in leprosy has been attributed to decreased number of functional melanocytes, reduced melanogenesis due to lack of Dopa oxidase activity or defective melanin transfer to keratinocytes [2].

The early lesions of LL are usually ill-defined macules which become slowly infiltrated and later present as papulo-nodules or diffuse infiltration. Hair loss is seen over the lesions mainly over the face manifesting as ciliary and super-ciliary madarosis. Sensation is usually unimpaired in the beginning but over the time, bilaterally symmetrical glove and stocking type of anesthesia can develop due to involvement of dermal nerves [3]. As the disease progresses, the peripheral nerve trunks become firm and hard.

Muscles of the hands and feet are affected directly as well as through the peripheral nerves resulting in weakness. Hands and feet may have swollen digits with tapering ends. Invasion of upper respiratory tract is common especially the nasal mucosa which can lead to nasal stuffiness and epistaxis. Hoarseness of voice results from laryngeal mucosa involvement. Eye changes in the form of corneal anesthesia, scleritis and episcleritis can occur and in the advanced stage, even blindness can occur [4].

Slit skin smear (SSS) in LL usually shows numerous AFB arranged in globi. Histopathology from skin lesion shows thin epidermis and clear Grenz zone. Dermis shows extensive infiltrate consisting of macrophages and foam cells along with few lymphocytes and plasma cells. AFB are seen in bundles like a pack of cigars or in large clumps called globi [5].

Differential diagnoses include Post Kala Azar Dermal leishmaniasis (PKDL), Cutaneous lymphoma and Sarcoidosis. PKDL, clinically characterized by hypo-pigmented macules, erythematous plaques and papulonodular lesions on the face extending to the other regions, can be differentiated from LL by involvement of muzzle area of face, sparing of ear lobes, absence of peripheral nerve thickening and loss of sensation, and also by the presence of Donovan bodies on histopathology [6]. Cutaneous Lymphomas can be ruled out by the presence of lymphadenopathy and organomegaly on clinical examination and atypical cells in peripheral blood smear. Sarcoidosis is differentiated by the absence of peripheral nerve thickening and loss of sensation, and also by the presence of well circumscribed granuloma devoid of collar of lymphocytes [5].

Treatment of Lepromatous Leprosy is with Rifampicin, Clofazamine and Dapsone in the form of MB-MDT (Multibacillary multi drug therapy) as directed by the world health organization (WHO). Untreated or inadequately treated cases may develop long term sequelae of nerve damage—atrophy of small muscles of hands and feet, trophic ulcer on weight bearing areas of the feet, loss of digits with absorption of terminal phalanges and autonomic disturbances among others [7].

Key Points
• The early lesions of LL are characterized by ill-defined hypopigmented macules being slowly infiltrated and ultimately present as diffuse infiltration or papules/nodules.

- Ciliary and supraciliary madarosis is another classical finding.
- Peripheral nerve thickening and bilateral glove and stocking anesthesia develop in advanced cases.
- Slit skin smears (SSS) showing multiple acid fast bacilli with Globi.

References

1. Kumar B, Dogra S. Leprosy: a disease with diagnostic and management challenges! Indian J Dermatol Venereol Leprol. 2009;75:111–5.
2. Kumar P, Savant SS, Das A. A curious case of lepromatous leprosy developing complete loss of pigmentation, followed by reappearance of pigmentation with multi drug therapy (MDT) alone—a support for neural theory of vitiligo pathogenesis? Indian J Lepr. 2018;90:155–9.
3. Madhusudan M. Leprous neuritis: a diagnostic dilemma. Indian J Dermatol Venereol Leprol. 1999;65:59–65.
4. Grzbowski A, Nita M, Virmond M. Ocular leprosy. Clin Dermatol. 2014;33:79–89.
5. Singh A, Ramesh V. Histopathological features in leprosy, post-kala-azar dermal leishmaniasis, and cutaneous leishmaniasis. Indian J Dermatol Venereol Leprol. 2013;79:360–6.
6. Arora S, D'Souza P, Haroon MA, Ramesh V, Kaur O, Chandoke RK. Post-kala-azar dermal leishmaniasis mimicking leprosy relapse: a diagnostic dilemma. Int J Dermatol. 2014;53:606–8.
7. Anand V, Pradhan S, Kumar P. Autonomic neuropathy impairing quality of life after completion of MDT: are we managing enough? Lepr Rev. 2016;87(2):239–42.

Part V
Reticulate Pigmentation

Chapter 20
A Young Female with Generalized Mottled Pigmentation

Swetalina Pradhan and Kananbala Sahu

A 20-year-old female presented with mottled pigmentation all over the body since her early childhood. There was no such history among family members. On close examination, there were both hypo and hyperpigmented macules of varying sizes being distributed over both trunk (Fig. 20.1) and extremities (Fig. 20.2).

From the above description and figure-diagnosis?

1. Reticulate acropigmentation of Dohi
2. Reticulate acropigmentation of Kitamura
3. Dyschromatosis universalis hereditaria
4. Dowling degos disease.

Histopathology of pigmented macules showed uniform increased pigment in epidermis with melanin incontinence.

Diagnosis

- Dyschromatosis universalis hereditaria

S. Pradhan (✉)
All India Institute of Medical Sciences, Patna, India

K. Sahu
All India Institute of Medical Sciences, Bhubaneswar, India

© Springer Nature Switzerland AG 2020   157
S. Kothiwala et al. (eds.), *Clinical Cases in Disorders of Melanocytes*, Clinical Cases in Dermatology,
https://doi.org/10.1007/978-3-030-22757-9_20

158   S. Pradhan and K. Sahu

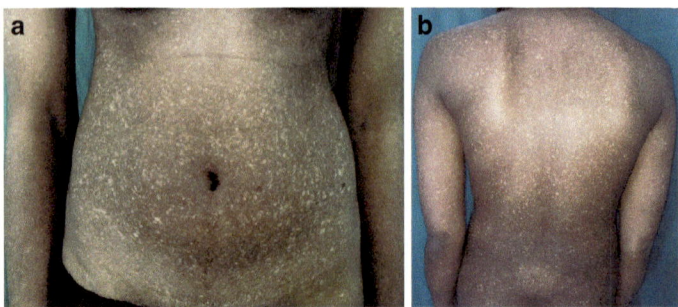

Figure 20.1 Mottled pigmentation over abdomen and back (Courtesy: Dr. Anup Kumar Tiwary)

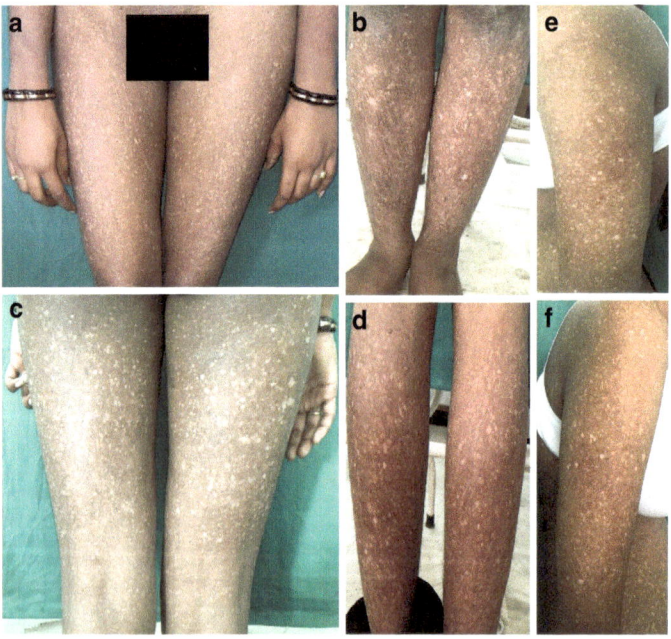

Figure 20.2 Similar lesions involving extremities (Courtesy: Dr. Anup Kumar Tiwary)

Discussion

Dyschromatosis universalis hereditaria (DUH) was originally believed to be a variant of localized acral form, dyschromatosis symmetrica hereditaria (DSH), also known as reticulate acropigmentation of Dohi [1]. Now a days, it seams to be different from dyschromatosis symmetrica hereditaria (DSH) with the genetic defect localized to 12q21-q23 loci [2]. It has mostly an autosomal dominant pattern of inheritance [3].

DUH starts in infancy or early childhood and is characterized by generalized mottled pigmentation. It starts from extremities and progress to involve the trunk and occasionally the face. The involvement of palm, soles and oral mucosa have also been reported in some cases [4]. The lesions are characterized by hyperpigmented macules admixed with hypopigmented macules of varying sizes. The nails are hyperpigmented and dystrophic with pterygium formation being the classic finding.

Various associations that have been reported include coxa valga, nerve compression, short stature, high-tone deafness, solar elastosis and neurosensory hearing defect.

Amyloidosis cutis dyschromia (ACD), DSH and xeroderma pigmentosum should always be considered as differential diagnosis of DUH. ACD is a very rare and distinctive variant of primary cutaneous amyloidosis, clinically characterized by the appearance of hyperpigmented and hypopigmented or depigmented macules on normal looking skin before puberty in generalized distribution [5]. DSH or reticulate acropigmentation of Dohi usually presents with mottled pigmentation over dorsa of hands and feet but may extend to proximal parts and face hence should be kept as differential. Xeroderma pigmentosum can be ruled out by characteristic involvement of photoexposed sites, skin atrophy, telangiectasia, photophobia and neoplastic changes with fatal course.

Besides the association, it is otherwise a benign condition which requires counselling of parents. Targeting the pigmented lesion with the Q-switched alexandrite laser is an option but recurrence is inevitable [6].

Key Points
- DUH is characterized by early life onset of hypopigmented and hyperpigmented macules of varying sizes all over body including covered area as well.
- Skin atrophy and telangiectasia are absent.
- There is no amyloid deposition in dermis.
- It runs a benign course.

References

1. Urabe K, Hori Y. Dyschromatosis. Semin Cutan Med Surg. 1997;16:81–5.
2. Suzuki N, Suzuki T, Inagaki K, Ito S, Kono M, Fukai K, et al. Mutation analysis of the ADAR1 gene in dyschromatosis symmetrica hereditaria and genetic differentiation from both dyschromatosis universalis hereditaria and acropigmentatio reticularis. J Invest Dermatol. 2005;124:1186–92.
3. Bolognia JL. Disorders of hypopigmentation and hyperpigmentation. In: Harper J, Orange H, Prose N, editors. Textbook of pediatric dermatology. 2nd ed. Hoboken: Blackwell Science; 2000. p. 868–70.
4. Ramrath K, Stolz W. Disorders of melanin pigmentation. In: Burgdorf W, Plewig G, Wolff HH, Landthaler M, editors. Braun Falco's dermatology. 3rd ed. New York: Springer; 2009. p. 772–4.
5. Tiwary AK, Mishra DK, Chaudhary SS. Amyloidosis cutis dyschromica: a rare dyschromic subtype of primary cutaneous amyloidosis. Pigment Int. 2016;3:33–6.
6. Nogita T, Mitsuhashi Y, Takeo C, Tsuboi R. Removal of facial and labial lentigines in dyschromatosis universalis hereditaria with a Q-switched alexandrite laser. J Am Acad Dermatol. 2011;65:61–3.

Chapter 21
A Female with Freckles Like Pigmentation on Face and Extremities

Swetalina Pradhan and Kananbala Sahu

A 24-year-old female presented with pigmentation over face and hands since her adolescent age. She also noticed gradual involvement of extensor of legs. The lesions were small, brown, depressed macules of <0.5 cm size. On close examination, there were well demarcated hyperpigmented macules on dorsum of hands, flexors of distal forearms (Figs. 21.1 and 21.2) and legs. Palm and sole had small pits with breaks in ridge pattern (Fig. 21.3). Similar lesions were also present in her mother.

From the above description and figure, what is the diagnosis?

1. Reticulate acropigmentation of Dohi
2. Reticulate acropigmentation of Kitamura
3. Dyschromatosis universalis hereditaria (DUH)
4. Dowling degos disease

Histopathology of pigmented macules showed epidermal atrophy and an increased number of basal melanocytes.

S. Pradhan (✉)
All India Institute of Medical Sciences, Patna, India

K. Sahu
All India Institute of Medical Sciences, Bhubaneswar, India

© Springer Nature Switzerland AG 2020
S. Kothiwala et al. (Eds.), *Clinical Cases in Disorders of Melanocytes*, Clinical Cases in Dermatology,
https://doi.org/10.1007/978-3-030-22757-9_21

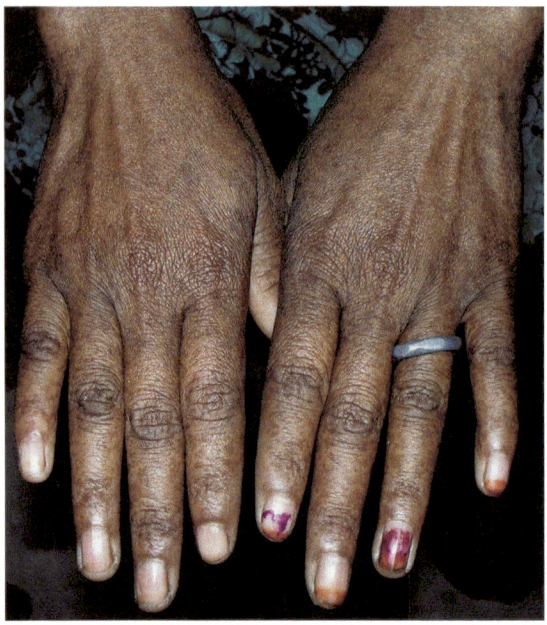

FIGURE 21.1 Well demarcated hyperpigmented macules on dorsum of hands (Courtesy: Dr. Piyush Kumar)

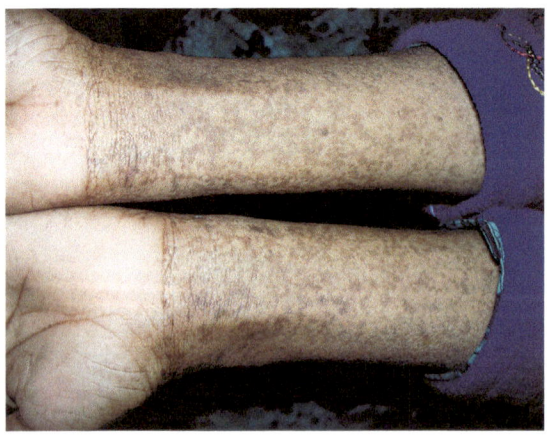

FIGURE 21.2 Similar lesions on flexors of distal forearms (Courtesy: Dr. Piyush Kumar)

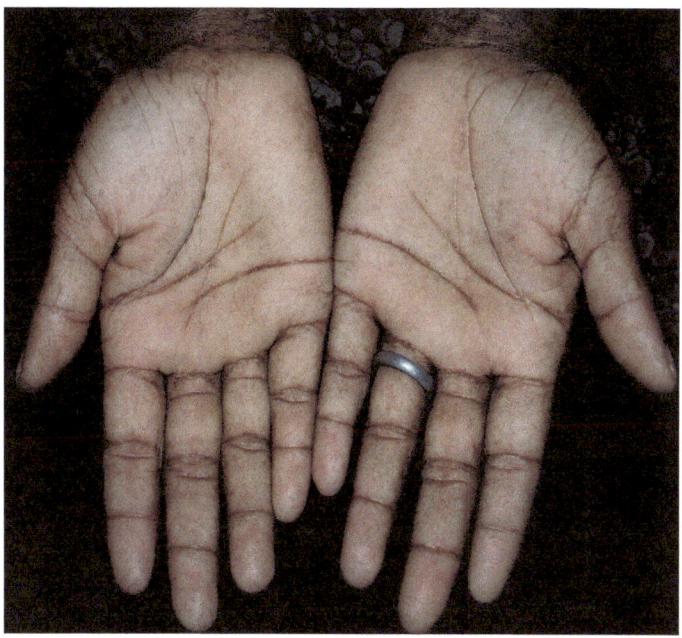

FIGURE 21.3 Palm and sole had small pits with breaks in ridge pattern (Courtesy: Dr. Piyush Kumar)

Diagnosis

• Reticulate acropigmentation of Kitamura

Discussion

Reticulate acropigmentation of Kitamura is an autosomal dominant condition mostly reported from the Asian countries [1]. There are a few reports of familial cases [2]. It occurs in first to second decade of life.

The lesions are slightly depressed, sharply demarcated black/brown macules localized to the dorsum of the hands and feet. The lesions increase in number and spread centripetally with age. The presence of small pits that cause a break in the epidermal ridge patterns on the palms and rarely on the dorsa of fingers is a diagnostic feature [1]. Eventually, the extensor aspects of the limbs, neck, upper trunk, face may be affected. The pigmentation may rarely extend to involve the flexures and the palms and soles. Uncommonly disseminated hypo- or depigmented macules and papules have also been reported. Histologically, hyperpigmented lesions show epidermal atrophy, elongation of rete ridges, and increased numbers of DOPA-positive melanocytes [3]. Differential diagnosis includes Dowling degos disease, reticulate acropigmentaation of Dohi and DUH.

Dowling degos disease is an autosomal dominant condition, also called as Dark dot disease, reticular pigmented anomaly of flexures [1]. This is characterized by spotted and reticulate pigmentation of the flexures, comedone-like papules on the back and neck and pitted perioral scars. It is usually sporadic though some affected families have been reported.

Reticulate acropigmentation of Dohi, also known as dyschromatosis symmetrica hereditaria (DSH) (autosomal dominant) begin in the first to second decade and are classically nonprogressive. It is characterized by hypo- and hyperpigmented macules on the dorsal aspect of hands and feet, which may extend to the proximal portion of the limbs. Sometimes, freckle-like macules can be found on the face [4]. The histology of the lesions shows either increased or decreased basilar pigmentation in the hyperpigmented or hypopigmented lesions respectively.

DUH has mostly infantile onset, characterized by generalized mottled pigmentation starting from extremities and progress to involve the trunk and occasionally the face [5]. The lesions are characterized by hyperpigmented macules admixed with hypopigmented macules of varying sizes. The nails are also hyperpigmented and dystrophic with pterygium formation.

Adapalene, systemic retinoids, azelaic acid and Q-switch alexandrite laser have been tried in a few patients with variable results.

Key Points
- Reticulate acropigmentation of Kitamura is an autosomal dominant condition mostly reported from the Asian countries, occurring in first to second decade of life.
- The classical lesions are slightly depressed, sharply demarcated black/brown macules localized to the dorsum of the hands and feet along with palmar pits.
- Rarely, face and trunk may also be involved.

References

1. James WD, Berger TG, Elston DM. Disturbances of pigmentation; pigmented anomalies of the extremities. Andrews' diseases of the skin clinical dermatology. 11th ed. China: Elsevier's; 2006. p. 855–6.
2. Kocatürk E, Kavala M, Zindanci I, Zemheri E, Koç MK, Sarigül S. Reticulate acropigmentation of Kitamura: report of a familial case. Dermatol Online J. 2008;14:7.
3. Kovarik CL, Spiehogel RL, Kantor GR. Pigmentary disorders of skin. In: Lever WF, Elder DE, editors. Lever's text book of histopathology. 2nd ed. New Delhi: Wolters Kluwer; 2009. p. 689–90.
4. Ramrath K, Stolz W. Disorders of melanin pigmentation. In: Burgdorf WH, Plewig G, Wolff HH, Landthaler M, editors. Braun Falco's dermatology. 3rd ed. New York: Springer; 2009. p. 772–4.
5. Bolognia JL. Disorders of hypopigmentation and hyperpigmentation. In: Harper J, Orange H, Prose N, editors. Textbook of pediatric dermatology. 2nd ed. Hoboken: Blackwell Science; 2000. p. 868–70.

Chapter 22
An Adult Male with Axillary Pigmentation

Avijit Mondal and Subhash Dasarathan

A 37-year-old male presented to the dermatology clinic with complaints of pigmentation in the axillae and groin for the past 15 years which was increasing gradually and was occasionally itchy. On close examination, it showed bilateral reticular pigmentation of axilla (Fig. 22.1), lower abdomen and upper part of thighs (Fig. 22.2). Lentigo-like and comedo-like lesions were also present over these areas. He denied any history of drug intake, intolerance to heat, decreased sweating, skin atrophy or involvement of extremities. There is history of similar lesions in his father.

Based on the case description and the photograph what is your diagnosis?

1. Acanthosis Nigricans
2. Neurofibromatosis
3. Dowling Degos disease
4. Reticulate pigmentation of Kitamura

Diagnosis

- Dowling Degos disease

A. Mondal (✉) · S. Dasarathan
College of Medicine and JNM Hospital, Kalyani, India

© Springer Nature Switzerland AG 2020   167
S. Kothiwala et al. (eds.), *Clinical Cases in Disorders of Melanocytes*, Clinical Cases in Dermatology,
https://doi.org/10.1007/978-3-030-22757-9_22

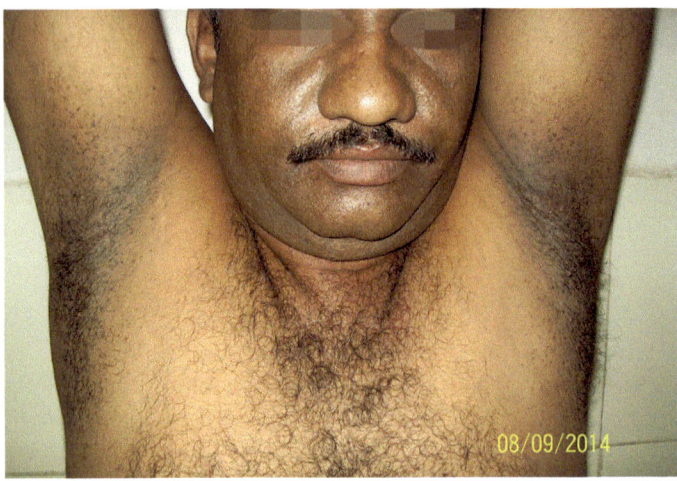

FIGURE 22.1 Reticular pigmentation of axilla (Courtesy: Dr. Santoshdev P Rathod)

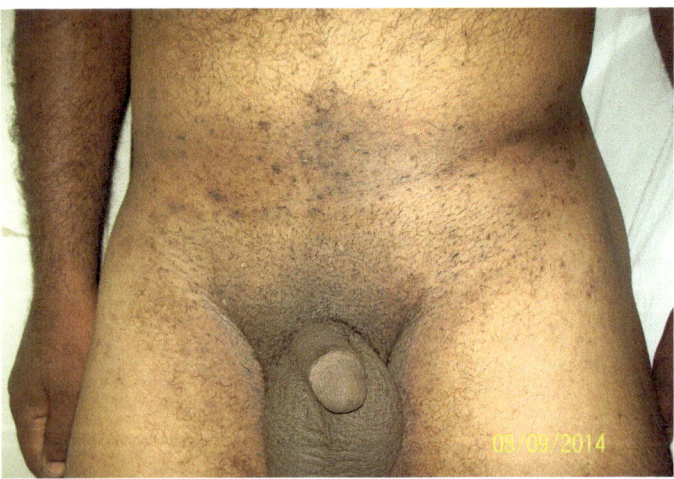

FIGURE 22.2 Lentigo-like and comedo-like lesions involving lower abdomen and thighs (Courtesy: Dr. Santoshdev P Rathod)

Discussion

Dowling Degos disease is a rare genetic disease of skin and is also known as reticulated pigmented anomaly of the flexures. It is an autosomal dominant condition with variable penetrance caused by the loss of function mutation in Keratin-5 gene which is involved in transfer of melanin from melanocytes to keratinocytes [1]. More recently it was found to be associated with POFUT1 gene (which encodes protein O-fucosyltransferase 1) and POGLUT1 gene (which encodes protein O-glucosyltransferase 1).

The onset is usually post-pubertal and is most common during the second to third decade of life. There seems to be a female predominance in reported cases. The pigmentation is reticular, progressive and disfiguring. The flexures are commonly involved with axillae and groin being the most common areas. It may be localized to one area like genital and perianal region (localized type) or gradually progressive to involve other areas (generalized type). The pigmentation may worsen in pregnancy and with sun exposure. Other cutaneous findings include comedo-like lesions over the neck and back, perioral pitted scars, epidermoid cysts and hidradenitis suppurativa. Hair and nails are not affected. A follicular variant has also been reported which is characterized by pigmented or non-pigmented raised scaly lesions based on follicle [2].

Diagnosis of DDD is made on the clinical features and confirmed by skin biopsy. Histologically, there is increased pigmentation of the basal layer, finger-like elongation of the rete ridges with suprapapillary thinning giving rise to an "antler like" pattern. Dermal melanophages and a mild perivascular lymphohistiocytic infiltrate can also be present [3].

Acanthosis nigricans, reticulate pigmentation of Kitamura and neurofibromatosis are the closest differential diagnosis. Acanthosis nigricans can be differentiated from Dowling degos disease clinically by velvety plaques and histologically by less pronounced elongation of rete ridges. Neurofibromatosis usually has multiple nodular lesions and Lisch nodules in the eyes. Reticulate pigmentation of Kitamura usually involves the extremities and presents with pigmented macules which are atrophic unlike Dowling Degos disease.

The best description of Dowling Degos disease was a mono letter mnemonic statement given by Wilson-Jones and Grice: Dusky Dappled Disfigurements and Dark Dot Depressions, and Disclosing Digitate Down growths Delving Dermally [4].

There is no successful treatment for DDD. Topical Steroids, retinoids and hydroquinone are used in treatment with varying success rates. Erbium: YAG laser has also been used [5].

Key Points
- Autosomal dominant Inheritance with mutation in Keratin 5 gene
- Postpubertal and young adults affected.
- Flexures (axillae and groin) are mostly affected.
- No satisfactory management.

References

1. Betz RC, Planko L, Eigelshoven S, et al. Loss-of-function mutations in the keratin 5 gene lead to Dowling-Degos disease. Am J Hum Genet. 2006;78:510–9.
2. Li C-R, Xing Q-H, Li M, et al. A gene locus responsible for reticulate pigmented anomaly of the flexures maps to chromosome 17p13.3. J Invest Dermatol. 2006;126:1297–301.
3. Kim YC, Davis MD, Schanbacher CF, Su WP. Dowling-Degos disease (reticulate pigmented anomaly of the flexures): a clinical and histopathologic study of 6 cases. J Am Acad Dermatol. 1999;40:462–7.
4. Rathoriya SG, Soni SS, Asati D. Dowling-Degos disease with reticulate acropigmentation of Kitamura: extended spectrum of a single entity. Indian Dermatol Online J. 2016;7(1):32–5.
5. Wenzel G, Petrow W, Tappe K. Treatment of Dowling-Degos disease with Er:YAG-laser: results after 2.5 years. Dermatol Surg. 2003;29:1161–2.

Part VI
Benign and Malignant Melanocytic Proliferation

Chapter 23
Deeply Pigmented Macules on Cheek and Neck

Anup Kumar Tiwary

A 12-year-old boy came in dermatology department present-ing with multiple, small, asymptomatic dark lesions on his right cheek and neck for past 2 years. The lesions appeared spontaneously without any history of trauma or dermatoses and have been static in size for past 1 year. The color remained same. No family history was present. On examination, there were three brown-black, well defined, macules of 3–4 mm size on right cheek (Fig. 23.1). Similar solitary brownish-black macule of about 4 × 3 mm size was noted on his neck on left side (Fig. 23.2). On dermoscopy, all lesions showed similar finding- multi-component pattern with peripheral reticular pigment network with blotchy pigmentation and pigmented globules in the centre (Fig. 23.3). Histopathology demon-strated nests of cuboidal melanocytes at the dermoepidermal junction, mainly located on the rete ridges.

What is the diagnosis?

1. Congenital melanocytic nevus
2. Junctional melanocytic nevus
3. Compound melanocytic nevus
4. Intradermal melanocytic nevus

———
A. K. Tiwary (✉)
Department of Dermatology, Subharti Medical College, Meerut, Uttar Pradesh, India

© Springer Nature Switzerland AG 2020   173
S. Kothiwala et al. (eds.), *Clinical Cases in Disorders of Melanocytes*, Clinical Cases in Dermatology,
https://doi.org/10.1007/978-3-030-22757-9_23

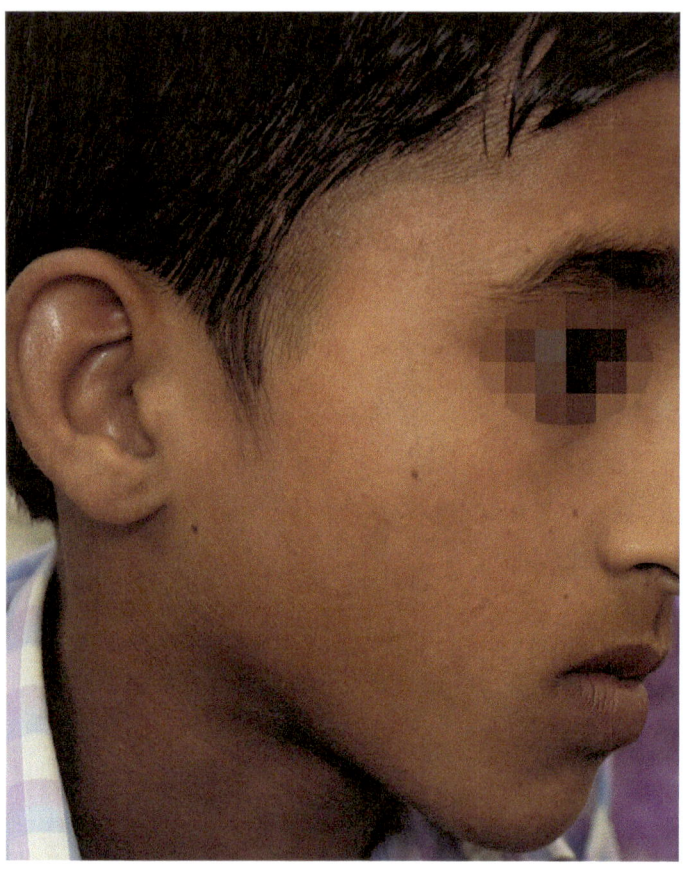

FIGURE 23.1 Deeply pigmented small size macules on right cheek
(Courtesy: Dr. Piyush Kumar)

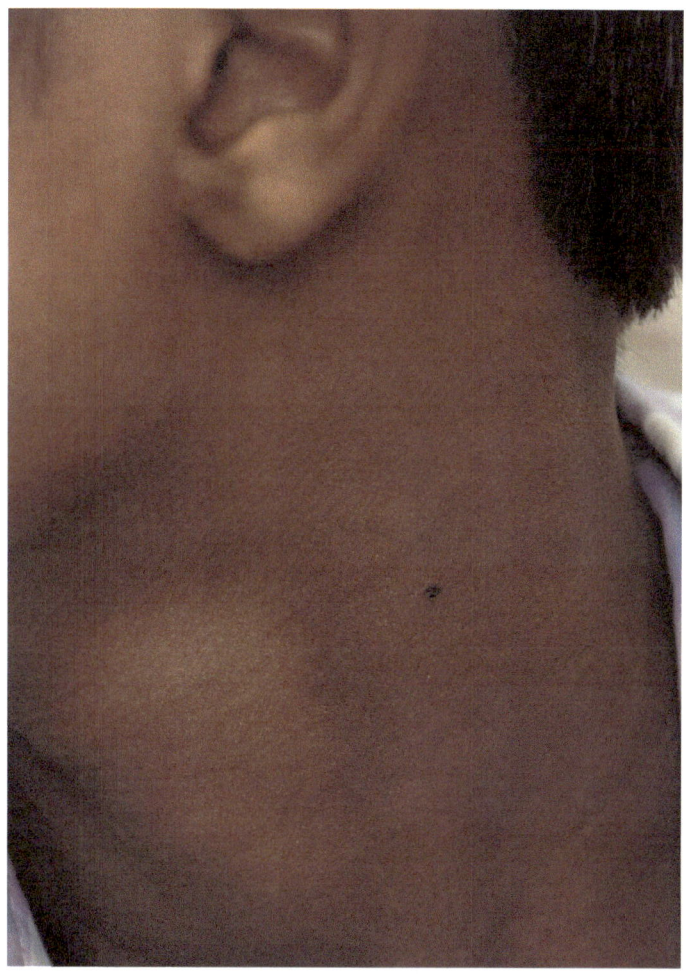

FIGURE 23.2 Deeply pigmented small size macule on neck (Courtesy: Dr. Piyush Kumar)

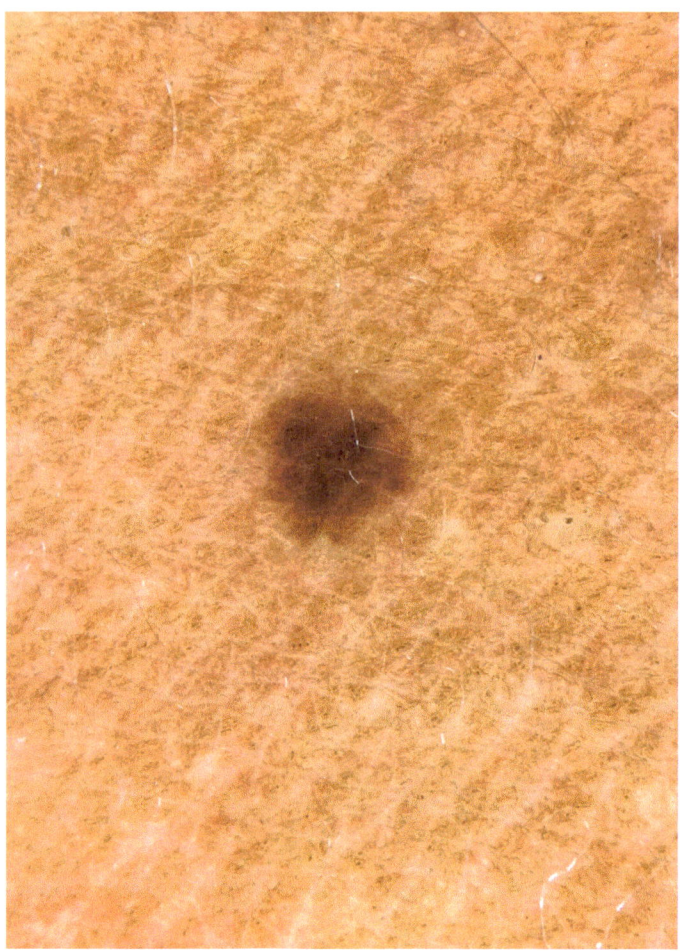

FIGURE 23.3 Dermoscopic image showing multi-component pattern with peripheral reticular pigment network with central blotchy pigmentation and pigmented globules (Courtesy: Dr. Piyush Kumar)

Diagnosis

- Junctional melanocytic nevus

Discussion

Junctional melanocytic nevus is one of the three common benign acquired melanocytic nevi (AMN)namely, junctional, compound and intradermal melanocytic nevus. These AMN are benign melanocytic proliferations mostly occurring in adults up to the age of about 40 years. In older age, it may either fade away or evolve into skin tag-like papules [1]. Aetiologically, it has been suggested that the mutation in BRAF oncogene (B-rapidly accelerated fibrosarcoma) leads to melanocytic neoplasia and UV rays may further aggravate the development of these nevi [2]. The evolution of AMN starts with the proliferation of melanocytes within the epidermis at the dermoepidermal junction, and therefore are known as junctional melanocytic nevi.

Junctional AMN are commonly seen in Fitzpatrick skin type I and II with no gender predilection. It usually presents as asymptomatic, brown/black, non-hairy macules (sometimes slightly elevated) mostly present on lateral aspect of arms, lower limbs, chest and back with tendency to remain small in size [3]. With time, nevus cells may 'drop down' into the dermis and undergo maturation and senescence, or neuroid differentiation. When the nevus cells are exclusively within the dermis, the nevi are known as dermal nevi. Risk of melanoma is rare. Dermoscopy of junctional AMN shows globular, reticular or mixed pattern. In young individuals, mixed central pattern is more common.

On histopathology, junctional nevi demonstrate the presence of theques of melanocytes that maintain contact with the basement membrane zone of the epidermis. Few melanocytes may sometimes be present higher within the epidermis. As the nevus matures, the melanocytes drop down into the dermis, become smaller and paler and form nests or cords [1].

Being a subtype of acquired AMN, junctional nevus has to be differentiated from other acquired AMN, compound and dermal. Junctional AMN may also simulate the clinical picture of congenital melanocytic nevi (CMN).

Dermal AMN are exclusively within the dermis and classically present as well marginated, dome-shaped skin-colored papule with single or multiple hairs emerging from the surface. It is mostly seen over face and upper back [1]. Individuals in second to fifth decade age group are mostly affected. Malignant changes are very rare.

Having both junctional and dermal elements, compound AMN present with combined features of junctional and dermal AMN. The compound nevus is round or oval and slowly becomes raised above the epidermal surface. The colour varies with the natural pigmentation of the patient and may be very dark, but the majority become paler with age [1]. There is usually little if any pigment on the flat surrounding epidermis. Limbs and back are common sites.

CMN is suggested to be caused by N-RAS or H-RAS (rat sarcoma oncogene) mutations, present at birth or develop in neonatal life [4]. Being much larger in diameter than acquired nevi, CMN is classified into three categories based on the diameter; small (<1.5 cm), medium (1.5–19.9 cm) and large (≥20 cm). The small/medium sized CMN appear as well-defined, light- to dark- brown macules or plaques with or without hypertrichosis. Of note, large/giant and older nevi often become palpable and develop deeply pigmented terminal hairs along with surface irregularities such as rugosites, mammillations or verrucous outgrowths simulating pigmented plexiform neurofibroma [5]. The presence of disseminated satellite nevi is another characteristic of giant CMN. Histopathology shows deep dermal nevomelanocytic cells with characteristic infiltration of adventitia of eccrine ducts, hair follicles, fat, smooth muscle, blood vessel walls and nerves. Giant CMN has significant risk of melanoma [6].

The junctional AMN can be left untreated with almost no risk of malignant changes, however the surgical excision can be done anytime to remove the lesion completely.

Key Points

- Junctional acquired benign melanocytic nevus usually presents as asymptomatic, brown/black, macules with no hairs
- The common sites are lateral aspect of arms, lower limbs, chest and back
- Fitzpatrick skin type I & II are more prone
- It usually remain small in size but nevus cells may go deep into the dermis and undergo maturation
- There is extremely rare chance of malignant transformation in junctional AMN

References

1. Newton-Bishop JA. Melanocytic naevi and melanoma. In: Hoeger PH, Yan AC, editors. Harper's textbook of pediatric dermatology. 3rd ed. Oxford: Wiley-Blackwell; 2011. p. 1242–3.
2. Wachsmuth RC, Turner F, Barrett JH, et al. The effect of sun exposure in determining nevus density in UK adolescent twins. J Invest Dermatol. 2005;124:56–62.
3. Richard MA, Grob JJ, Gouvernet J, et al. Role of sun exposure on nevus. First study in age-sex phenotype-controlled populations. Arch Dermatol. 1993;129:1280–5.
4. Dessars B, de Raeve LE, Morandini R, et al. Genotypic and gene expression studies in congenital melanocytic nevi: insight into initial steps of melanotumorigenesis. J Invest Dermatol. 2009;129:139–47.
5. Strauss RM, Newton-Bishop JA. Spontaneous involution of congenital melanocytic nevi of the scalp. J Am Acad Dermatol. 2008;58:508–11.
6. Swerdlow AJ, English JS, Qiao Z. The risk of melanoma in patients with congenital nevi: a cohort study. J Am Acad Dermatol. 1995;32:595–9.

Chapter 24
Solitary Pigmented Skin Lesion with Surrounding Loss of Pigmentation

Anup Kumar Tiwary

A 20-year-old female presented with a pigmented solid elevated lesion surrounded by white discoloration on her neck for past 4 years. It was completely asymptomatic. On close cutaneous examination, there was a central black papule on left upper region of neck, of size 0.7 cm in diameter with regular border. It was surrounded by a complete depigmented halo which was oval and regular in shape and about 3 cm in its maximum dimension (Fig. 24.1). No personal or family history of similar lesion was noted. Histopathology of central papule revealed nevomelanocytic proliferations and dense dermal lymphocytic infiltrates. Based on clinico-histopathologic details and image, what is your diagnosis?

1. Mayerson's nevus
2. Cockade nevus
3. Halo nevus
4. Regressing melanoma

A. K. Tiwary (✉)
Department of Dermatology, Subharti Medical College, Meerut, Uttar Pradesh, India

© Springer Nature Switzerland AG 2020   181
S. Kothiwala et al. (eds.), *Clinical Cases in Disorders of Melanocytes*, Clinical Cases in Dermatology,
https://doi.org/10.1007/978-3-030-22757-9_24

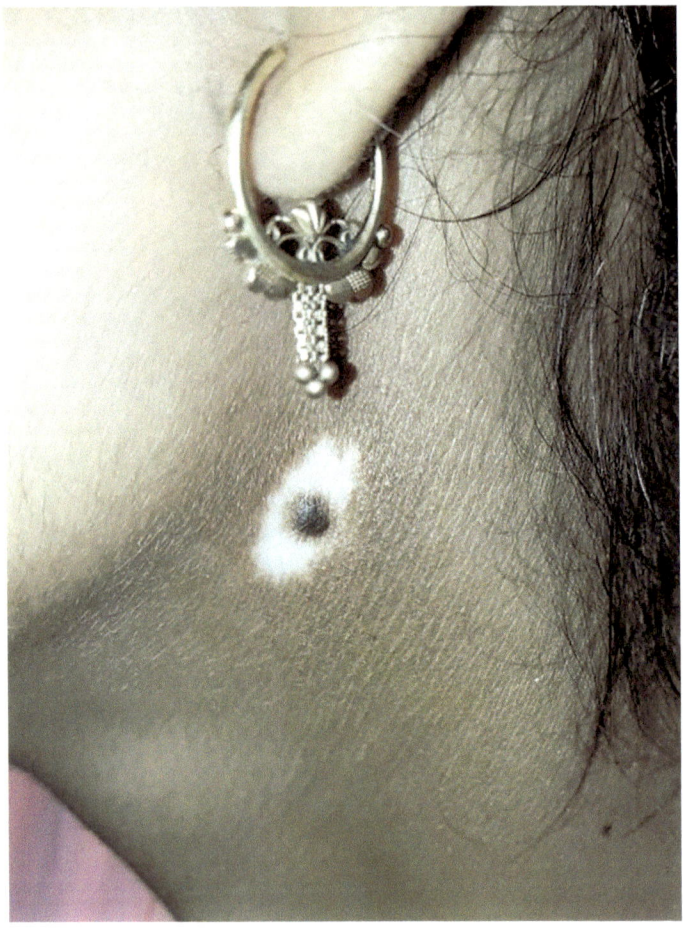

FIGURE 24.1 Solitary pigmented papule on neck surrounded by depigmented skin

Diagnosis

• Halo nevus

Discussion

Halo nevus, synonymously known as Sutton's nevus, perinevoid vitiligo, and leukoderma acquisitum centrifugum, is a melanocytic nevus surrounded by a rim of hypopigmentation or depigmentation [1]. It tends to be multiple in number and usually affects individuals in second decade of life with no gender or racial predilection. The commonest site is upper back followed by neck and abdomen. The central nevus may partially or completely regress in years with or without repigmentation of halo [2].

The development of halo is thought to result from host's immunologic reactions, chiefly consisting of inflammatory cytokines and cytotoxic CD8+ T cells [3]. The finding of elevated circulating antibodies against melanocytic antigens is only secondary to the destruction of melanocytes.

The typical halo nevus presents as solitary or multiple, darkly pigmented, benign compound melanocytic nevus with a surrounding symmetric, well-defined, rim of depigmented zone. The central papule as well as peripheral halo, both have regular borders. In white skin, it is more appreciable during the summer months showing the non-tanned halo in sharp contrast to the normal skin. The diameter of the halo is correlated to the size of the central nevus, the larger the nevus, the larger the halo. Halo nevi are also associated with vitiligo and a vitiligo-like phenomenon. Approximately 20% of individuals with halo nevi have vitiligo.

Histopathologically, the nevus may be junctional, compound or dermal, with dense lymphocytic infiltrates surrounding or permeating the dermal component. The nevus cells may become vacuolated with pyknotic nuclei [4]. The use of DOPA stains usually reveal a loss of epidermal melanocytes in the halo area. The peripheral white halo has little or no lymphocytic infiltrate. Regression of the central nevus is not associated with fibrosis, in contrast to the regression of melanoma, due to increased levels of antifibrotic tumor necrosis factor (TNF)-α.

Mayerson's nevus, cockade nevus and regressing melanoma are usually included in close differential diagnosis of halo nevus.

Mayerson's nevus: It is clinically presented by a melanocytic nevus developing surrounding eczematous inflammatory reaction associated with epidermal scaling and pruritus. It is usually solitary, but can be multiple and nearly three times as common in males compared to females. The trunk is the most common site, although any site can be affected. Unlike in halo nevus, Meyerson's nevus does not regress. The histopathology is usually that of an acquired melanocytic nevus with associated spongiotic dermal dermatitis predominated by CD4+ T-lymphocytes that miss other markers of T helper cells such as BCL-6 or CD10 [5].

Cockade nevus: It is a rare variant of acquired melanocytic nevus that peculiarly presents as a target-like nevi, resembling a rosette [6]. There is a hypochromic zone between pigmented central junctional melanocytic nevus and pigmented halo, giving it a target-like configuration. These are usually multiple in number and affect young people. Spinal dysraphism and juvenile diabetes mellitus are its known associations. On histopathology, it does not show cellular infiltrates unlike in halo nevus.

Melanoma: Being an immunogenic tumor and infiltrated by high levels of T lymphocytes, the course of melanoma may witness spontaneous regression with pigmentary changes. It may be clinically evident as depigmentation either within a melanocytic lesion, around melanocytic nevi (halo nevi) or in a distant site (melanoma-associated depigmentation) [7]. Of these, 'melanoma with a depigmented halo' simulate the picture of benign halo nevus. Of note, the halo of melanoma is more irregular than that seen in halo nevus and the patients are usually older. To add, histopathology of melanoma with halo during regression reveals fibrous stroma replacing the dermal portion of the tumor [8].

Excisional biopsy is the best recommendation to rule out the possibility of malignancy. However, it can be left keeping under observation.

Key Points

- Halo nevus presents as darkly pigmented melanocytic nevus with a surrounding well-defined rim of depigmented skin.
- The central nevus may partially or completely regress in years with or without repigmentation of halo.
- Regression of the central nevus is not associated with fibrosis unlike in melanoma.

References

1. Rados J, Pastar Z, Lipozencic J, Ilic I, Stulhofer Buzina D. Halophenomenon with regression of acquired melanocytic nevi: a case report. Acta Dermatovenerol Croat. 2009;17:139–43.
2. Aouthmany M, Weinstein M, Zirwas MJ, Brodell RT. The natural history of halo nevi: a retrospective case series. J Am Acad Dermatol. 2012;67:582–6.
3. Moretti S, Spallanzani A, Pinzi C, Prignano F, Fabbri P. Fibrosis in regressing melanoma versus nonfibrosis in halo nevus upon melanocyte disappearance: could it be related to a different cytokine microenvironment? J Cutan Pathol. 2007;34:301–8.
4. Akasu R, From L, Kahn HJ. Characterization of the mononuclear infiltrate involved in regression of halo nevi. J Cutan Pathol. 1994;21:302–11.
5. Wollina U. Nevi presenting a halo: Sutton nevus, Meyerson nevus, and Wollina-Schaarschmidt halo-like dermatosis. Our Dermatol Online. 2017;8(2):149–51.
6. Mehregan AH, King JR. Multiple target-like pigmented nevi. Arch Dermatol. 1972;105:129–30.
7. Naveh HP, Rao UN, Butterfield LH. Melanoma-associated leukoderma—immunology in black and white? Pigment Cell Melanoma Res. 2013;26(6):796–804.
8. Rubegni P, Nami N, Risulo M, Tataranno D, Fimiani M. Melanoma with halo. Clin Exp Dermatol. 2009;34:749–50.

Chapter 25
Solitary Nonhealing Noduloulcerative Lesion on Heel of Left Foot

Anup Kumar Tiwary and Sunil Kumar Kothiwala

A 57-year-old male came to dermatology OPD with solitary tender pigmented and thickened skin lesion on left sole for past 2 years. The color was appreciated as bluish-black and the whole skin lesion was about 6.5 cm in its greatest dimension. On close examination, a plaque of size 2.5 × 5 cm with a small oval ulcer was noted. This plaque had a lateral continuation consisting of macular component of same color (Fig. 25.1). It started as painless flat blue-black lesion which later on evolved into plaque and developed ulcer. There was no pre-existing skin lesion and no such family history was noted. Systemic examinations were unremarkable and there was no lymphadenopathy.

Based on the case description and photographs, what is the diagnosis?

1. Acral junctional nevus
2. Talon noir
3. Ulcerative lichen planus
4. Acral lentiginous melanoma

A. K. Tiwary (✉)
Department of Dermatology, Subharti Medical College, Meerut, Uttar Pradesh, India

S. K. Kothiwala
Dr. Kothiwala's SkinEva Clinic, Jaipur, India

© Springer Nature Switzerland AG 2020
S. Kothiwala et al. (eds.), *Clinical Cases in Disorders of Melanocytes*, Clinical Cases in Dermatology,
https://doi.org/10.1007/978-3-030-22757-9_25

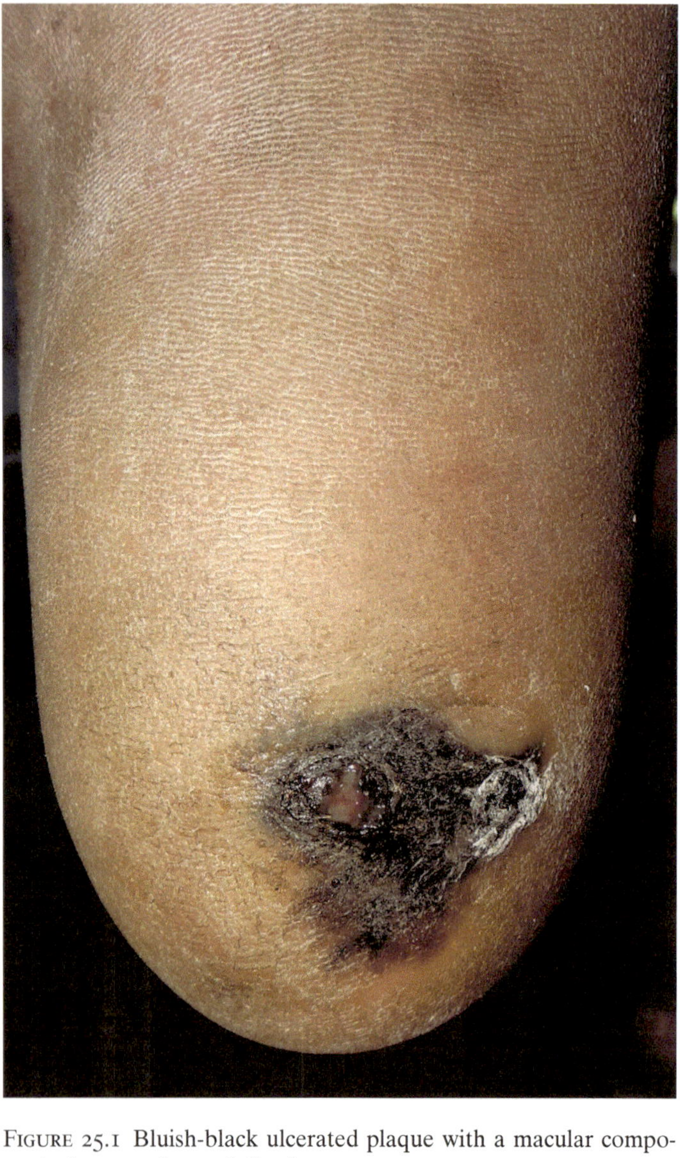

FIGURE 25.1 Bluish-black ulcerated plaque with a macular component of same color on left sole

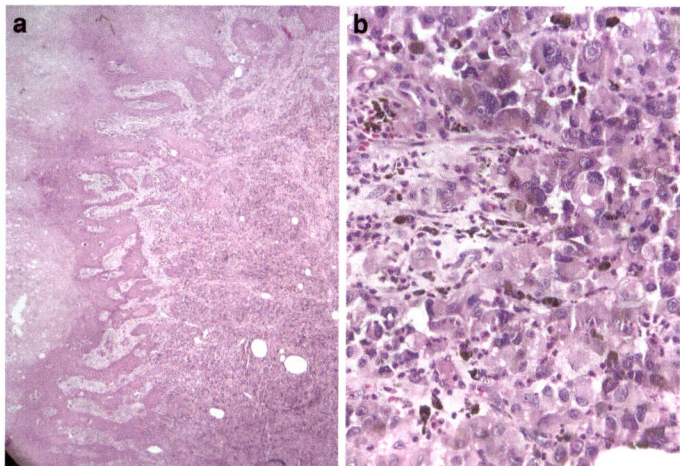

FIGURE 25.2 (**a**) Epidermal acanthosis, diffusely present pigment in stratum corneum and acrosyrinx, single-cell melanocytic proliferation along dermo-epidermal junction, lymphocytic infiltrates and spindle cells in dermis (H&E ×40). (**b**) Higher magnification (H&E ×400)

Histopathologic examination revealed epidermal acanthosis, diffusely present pigment in stratum corneum and acrosyrinx, single-cell melanocytic proliferation along dermo-epidermal junction, lymphocytic infiltrates and spindle cells in dermis (Fig. 25.2a, b).

Diagnosis

• Acral lentiginous melanoma

Discussion

Melanoma is one of the most common malignant skin tumor with wide ethnic variations. It has four common types namely, superficial spreading, nodular, lentigo maligna and acral lentiginous melanoma (ALM), with first one being most common type in white people. Of note, ALM is commonest in skin of color (Blacks, Asians, and Hispanics) accounting for 35–60% of melanomas having more advanced disease and poorer prognosis [1]. As the name suggests, it involves acral regions preferentially palms and soles. Elderly people are commonly affected and the incidence varies from 1 to 2 per million per year.

Aetiologically, occurrence of ALM has been attributed to some environmental triggering factors in genetically predisposed individuals. These external risk factors are trauma (especially burn and penetrating injuries), chemical exposure, tobacco use, pre-existing dysplastic nevi and malignant skin tumors [2]. Sunlight has no contribution unlike in other forms of melanoma. In most of the cases, mutations in BRAF, NRAS, MEK, ERK and wild-type KIT have been reported that lead to dysregulated mitogen-activated protein kinase (MAPK) pathway [3].

ALM was first described by RJ Reed in 1976 as pigmented lesions on the extremities, particularly on plantar regions characterized by an initial lentiginous/radial growth phase evolving with time to a late dermal/invasive phase [1]. Other common sites are palmar surface of the hands, fingers, toes and subungual region [4]. ALM usually starts with darkly pigmented blue-black macules (majority have >7 mm diameter) with irregular margins. Over the time, it becomes plaque with elevation of central area and at this stage, it is simulated by non-healing traumatic wounds, warts, chronic paronychia and pyogenic granulomas. Over months or years it evolves into tender nodules or exophytic lesions. Ulceration and bleeding are poor clinical prognostic signs.

Acral junctional nevus, talon noir and ulcerated lichen planus (LP) must be ruled out in all such cases. Acral junctional nevus potentially shares the clinical similarities, especially with early stage of ALM. It mostly presents as flat, dark brown macule with irregular border and of size usually ranging from 0.3 to 10 mm depending upon site and ethnicity of people [5]. It runs a benign course and histopathology is essential to rule out melanoma. Talon noir is one of the closest differentials of ALM which is caused due to traumatic rupture of dermal capillaries leading to intraepidermal haemorrhage. It presents as asymptomatic, bilaterally distributed violet-black macules on the heels, head of metatarsals, palms and fingers [6]. Paring reveals puncta of the black pigment of extravasated red cells confirming the diagnosis of talon noir. Ulcerative LP usually starts as erythema and bullae on the sole which runs a chronic and progressive course ultimately resulting in ulcers, scarring and deformities [7].

Early clinical diagnosis of ALM is essential and dermoscopy patterns help in determining accurate diagnosis of ALM. In the early phase of ALM dermoscopic findings are more useful than histopathological findings. The most important dermoscopic features of ALM are:

1. Parallel ridge pattern—It is most important dermoscopy findings and can be easily observed as pigment distribution along the ridges of skin. The sensitivity and specificity for ALM are 86.4% and 99%, respectively [8]
2. Asymmetry of color and structure
3. Blue gray structures
4. A linear and haphazard distribution of acrosyringia.

Features of benign melanocytic lesions like parallel-furrow pattern, lattice like pattern, or fibrillar pattern may also be present, but they are focal and found in association with parallel ridge pattern. Dermoscopy of subungual ALM shows a brown background with longitudinal irregular lines. Another specific finding is triangular shape of the band that represents enlargement of the proximal edge of the longitudinal melanonychia.

In a suspicious case of ALM, it is best cut out. A partial or punch biopsy could miss a focus of melanoma arising in pre-existing nevus, so it is best avoided except in unusually large lesions. Early lesions show presence of tumor cells in single unit that later coalesce into nests. The nests in ALM are non-cohesive, variable sized, poorly circumscribed and located parallel to the epidermis in contrast to melanocytic nevus where they are cohesive, similar in size, well circumscribed and located vertically. Some of the tumor cells can be present in the upper layer of epidermis in both melanocytic nevus and ALM. In malenocytic nevus, the tumor cells ascent along furrow. But in ALM, they tend to ascend along ridges which show consistency with the dermoscopic findings. To catch these histopathological findings making perpendicular sections to the ridges and furrows is essential. The nuclei of melanocytic nevus are usually smaller than those of the adjacent keratinocytes, so when nuclei of tumor cell are larger than keratinocytes, possibility of ALM should be considered. Thick and long dendrites reaching up to upper layers of epidermis favors malignancy hence HMB45 immunostaining is useful to assess the dendrite shape [9]. Diagnosing early subungual ALM histopathologically is often challenging. Increased number of melanocytes (>30 tumor cells in 1-mm width of epidermis) is an important finding that favors malignancy over benign nevus, although some malignant lesions may show low cellularity. Therefore clinical information and dermoscopic findings are essential for diagnosis of ALM.

The initial treatment of a primary ALM is to cut it out; the lesion should be completely excised with a 2–3 mm margin of normal tissue. Further treatment depends mainly on the Breslow thickness of the lesion. The radial excision margins, measured clinically from the edge of the melanoma and it range from 5 mm for melanoma in-situ to 2 cm for melanoma with >4.0 mm thickness. After surgical excision, primary closure, skin grafting, secondary intension healing, and local and free flaps are performed based on size of wound and site. As ALM frequently occurs on sole, a full thickness skin graft is often used when primary closure is impossible. Surgical excision is challenging in subungual ALM because of the close distance between nail and underlying bone. Conservative surgery with excision at the level of distal phalanx in in-situ and wide excision with phalanx amputation for thick subungual ALM may be done.

Melanoma staging helps in deciding the approach to manage the melanoma which has spread from its original site in the skin. Staging recommended by American Joint Committee on Cancer (AJCC) cutaneous melanoma staging guidelines (2009) are widely acceptable.

- Stage 0—In situ melanoma
- Stage 1—Thin melanoma <2 mm in thickness
- Stage 2—Thick melanoma >2 mm in thickness
- Stage 3—Melanoma spread to involve local lymph nodes
- Stage 4—Distant metastases have been detected

If the local lymph nodes are enlarged, they should be removed. If lymph nodes are not enlarged, they may be tested microscopically to see presence of tumor cells. The presence or absence of tumor cells in sentinel lymph nodes (SLN) is well known to be an independent factor for the prognosis so SLN biopsy is now recommended in melanoma patients with intermediate-thickness tumors. In a recent study, ALM showed the highest frequency of positive SLNs [10].

If the melanoma is widespread, other forms of treatment may be necessary, but are not always successful in eradicating the cancer. The response rate for immune check point inhibitors is low for ALM in comparison to other types of melanoma. Chemotherapy with dacarbazine (DTIC), imiquimod, interferons, biologics such as ipilimumab, and BRAF inhibitors such as vemurafenib and dabrafenib are showing promise. Follow-up visits are required to check scar and regional lymph nodes to detect early recurrence.

Key Points
- Acral lentiginous melanoma is the commonest type of melanoma in people of color mostly affecting palmoplantar area.
- It has more aggressive course and poorer prognosis than other types.
- Any acquired darkly pigmented irregularly marginated macule or plaque of size >7 mm on sole or palm in an elderly people should always be biopsied to rule out ALM.
- Diffusely present pigment in stratum corneum and around acrosyrinx, single-cell atypical melanocytic proliferation along dermo-epidermal junction, lymphocytic infiltrates and spindle cells and/or pagetoid cells in dermis are characteristic histopathologic features.

- Determination of patterns on dermoscopy is essential for accurate diagnosis of ALM.
- ALM patients may show shorter survival because it shows less susceptibility to immune checkpoint inhibitors and less frequent BRAF mutations.

References

1. Bradford PT, Goldstein AM, McMaster ML, Tucker MA. Acrallentiginous melanoma: incidence and survival patterns in the United States, 1986-2005. Arch Dermatol. 2009;145(4):427–34.
2. Liu XK, Li J. Acral lentiginous melanoma. Lancet. 2018;391:e21.
3. Bastian BC. The molecular pathology of melanoma: an integrated taxonomy of melanocytic neoplasia. Annu Rev Pathol. 2014;9:239–71.
4. Piliang MP. Acral lentiginous melanoma. Clin Lab Med. 2011;31(2):2818.
5. Palicka GA, Rhodes AR. Acral melanocytic nevi: prevalence and distribution of gross morphologic features in white and black adults. Arch Dermatol. 2010;146(10):1085–94.
6. Keerthi S, Madhavi S, Karthikeyan K. Talon noir: a mirage of melanoma. Pigment Int. 2015;2:54–6.
7. Hassan S, Das A, Kumar P. Solitary painful ulcerated plaque on the sole. Indian Dermatol Online J. 2015;6:131–3.
8. Saida T, Miyazaki A, Oguchi S, Ishihara Y, Yamazaki Y, Murase S, et al. Significance of dermoscopic patterns in detecting malignant melanoma on acral volar skin: results of a multicenter study in Japan. Arch Dermatol. 2004;140(10):1233–8.
9. Nakamura Y, Fujusawa Y. Diagnosis and management of acral lentiginous melanoma. Curr Treat Options in Oncol. 2018;19:42–53.
10. Marek AJ, Ming ME, Bartlett EK, Karakousis GC, Chu EY. Acral lentiginous histologic subtype and sentinel lymph node positivity in thin melanoma. JAMA Dermatol. 2016;152(7):836–7.

Index

© Springer Nature Switzerland AG 2020
S. Kothiwala et al. (eds.), *Clinical Cases in Disorders of Melanocytes*, Clinical Cases in Dermatology,
https://doi.org/10.1007/978-3-030-22757-9